More Praise for Dr. Sari Fine Shepphird
Answers About Anorexia Nervosa

100 Questions and Answers About Anorexia Nervosa is full of good information. It is practical and easy to read and it answers many of the most frequently asked questions in an easy to understand, non-judgmental, and straightforward way. It should be on the bookshelf of every high school and public library in the country; it should be made available to all clinicians, educators, and community members who work with youth. Parents and loved ones should be given a copy when they are just beginning the journey into recovery from anorexia. Thank you Dr. Shepphird!

> Excerpt from the Foreword by **Kitty Westin**
> *Founder, Anna Westin Foundation*
> *(now the Emily Program Foundation)*
> *President, Eating Disorders Coalition for Research, Policy & Action*

Comprehensive, solid, detailed, very well researched, and well written, *100 Questions and Answers About Anorexia Nervosa* provides the most up to date treatment approaches and explains clearly what individuals and families should know in trying to find treatment for themselves or their loved one. The emphasis here is on realistic, positive solutions. The author has a masterful command of this serious illness and through questions and detailed answers, Dr. Shepphird gives the reader a vast fund of knowledge, and most importantly hope, in tackling and resolving this disorder at a personal level.

> **Richard Sherman, PhD**
> *Clinical Psychologist, Tarzana, California*
> *Past President, California Psychological Association*

An extremely enlightening book, *100 Questions and Answers About Anorexia Nervosa* is going to be a wonderful resource for eating disorder patients and their families. It is easy to read, very informative, and goes over many of the most common questions that are asked by people about anorexia nervosa and eating disorders with added beneficial information.

> **Ellen Reiss-Goldfarb, RD**
> *Registered Dietitian and Nutrition Therapist*
> *Los Angeles, California*

100 Questions & Answers About Anorexia Nervosa

Sari Fine Shepphird, PhD
Clinical Psychologist
Eating Disorders Specialist
Los Angeles, California

JONES AND BARTLETT PUBLISHERS
Sudbury, Massachusetts
BOSTON   TORONTO   LONDON   SINGAPORE

World Headquarters

Jones and Bartlett Publishers	Jones and Bartlett Publishers	Jones and Bartlett Publishers
40 Tall Pine Drive	Canada	International
Sudbury, MA 01776	6339 Ormindale Way	Barb House, Barb Mews
978-443-5000	Mississauga, Ontario L5V 1J2	London W6 7PA
info@jbpub.com	Canada	United Kingdom
www.jbpub.com		

Jones and Bartlett's books and products are available through most bookstores and online booksellers. To contact Jones and Bartlett Publishers directly, call 800-832-0034, fax 978-443-8000, or visit our website, www.jbpub.com.

Substantial discounts on bulk quantities of Jones and Bartlett's publications are available to corporations, professional associations, and other qualified organizations. For details and specific discount information, contact the special sales department at Jones and Bartlett via the above contact information or send an email to specialsales@jbpub.com.

The authors, editor, and publisher have made every effort to provide accurate information. However, they are not responsible for errors, omissions, or for any outcomes related to the use of the contents of this book and take no responsibility for the use of the products and procedures described. Treatments and side effects described in this book may not be applicable to all people; likewise, some people may require a dose or experience a side effect that is not described herein. Drugs and medical devices are discussed that may have limited availability controlled by the Food and Drug Administration (FDA) for use only in a research study or clinical trial. Research, clinical practice, and government regulations often change the accepted standard in this field. When consideration is being given to use of any drug in the clinical setting, the healthcare provider or reader is responsible for determining FDA status of the drug, reading the package insert, and reviewing prescribing information for the most up-to-date recommendations on dose, precautions, and contraindications, and determining the appropriate usage for the product. This is especially important in the case of drugs that are new or seldom used.

Production Credits

Senior Acquisitions Editor: Alison Hankey	VP, Manufacturing and Inventory Control:
Sr. Editorial Assistant: Jessica Acox	Therese Connell
Production Director: Amy Rose	Composition: Appingo Publishing Services
Production Assistant: Laura Almozara	Printing and Binding: Malloy, Inc.
Marketing Manager: Ilana Goddess	Cover Printing: Malloy, Inc.

Cover Credits
Cover Design: Carolyn Downer
Cover Images: Top left: © Jason Stitt/ShutterStock, Inc.; Top right: © Andresr/ShutterStock, Inc.; Bottom left: © Yuri Arcurs/ShutterStock, Inc.; Bottom right: © Christopher Halloran/ShutterStock, Inc.

Library of Congress Cataloging-in-Publication Data

Shepphird, Sari Fine.
  100 questions and answers about anorexia nervosa / Sari Fine Shepphird.
    p. cm.
  Includes bibliographical references and index.
  ISBN-13: 978-0-7637-5450-1
  ISBN-10: 0-7637-5450-1
  1. Anorexia nervosa—Miscellanea. 2. Eating disorders—Miscellanea. 3. Teenage girls—Mental health—Miscellanea. 4. Body image in adolescence—Miscellanea. I. Title. II. Title: One hundred questions and answers about anorexia nervosa.
  RC552.A5S54 2009
  616.85'262—dc22
                                            2008038717

6048
Printed in the United States of America
13 12 11 10 09   10 9 8 7 6 5 4 3 2

To my great-grandparents—
for the possibilities.

CONTENTS

Questions 1–11 give background information about anorexia nervosa and discuss such topics as:

- What is anorexia nervosa?
- How is the diagnosis of anorexia determined?
- Is anorexia dangerous? What are the risks associated with anorexia?
- Do people with anorexia get better?

Questions 12–21 outline the characteristic signs and symptoms of anorexia nervosa as well as related issues, including:

- What is "starvation syndrome"?
- Before my son developed anorexia, I thought it was only a problem for girls. What are some other myths about anorexia?
- It seems like there are many reasons why a person might lose appetite and not eat for a period of time. How can one know if anorexia is the cause?

Questions 22–27 discuss the causes and risk factors for developing anorexia, including:

- What causes anorexia nervosa?
- How does the mass media influence ideas about anorexia and eating disorders?

Contents

I have no doubt that you, like I, have questions about anorexia (a complicated and confusing illness) and have been searching for answers. "What is anorexia nervosa?" "My daughter recently said she just wanted to 'lose a little weight' in order to feel better about herself. Should I be concerned?" "I know that caring for my daughter will be a challenge, but I'm not sure what to expect. What type of difficulties might I face?" These questions, and so many more, are answered in *100 Questions and Answers About Anorexia Nervosa*, written by eating disorder treatment expert Dr. Sari Shepphird. Some of the questions have fairly simple answers, and others are very complex and complicated; but all are worthy, need to be addressed, and deserve thoughtful, straightforward answers.

"What do I want?" "Where has my ability and confidence gone?" "How can I get through this, and will I ever feel good again?" These are questions Anna Westin (1978–2000) wrote in her diary while she was fighting anorexia.

"How did this happen?" "What can I do to help?" "Will she recover?" These are some of the questions I had when my daughter, Anna Westin, was fighting anorexia.

I vividly recall the day I sat with my husband Mark and our daughter Anna in an office at a local hospital and heard the diagnosis: Anna had anorexia nervosa, a serious and potentially fatal illness if left untreated. I was stunned, and I don't recall much else that was said except: "Anna needs immediate hospitalization or she will die." It took my breath away. I looked over at Mark, and he had tears in his eyes; I looked at Anna, and she was staring back at me blankly. That's the moment I knew we were in for the fight of our lives—literally, the fight for Anna's life. I had so many questions but did not know where to begin or even who to ask. I felt helpless and alone. I wondered why I was not able to protect my daughter and keep her safe. I was sure I had failed her and that I must have done something wrong. My heart broke that day.

Anna was first diagnosed with anorexia when she was 16 years old. She went into treatment and seemed to fully recover, and I was certain that her life was back on track. She had so much potential; dreams, goals, and a lifetime filled with love and joy to look forward to. I never dreamed an eating disorder would sneak back into her life 5 years later and within months take her from us.

In retrospect, I ask myself these questions: How was I to know that Anna's nearly impossibly high standards for herself and her need for structure and order could have been early warning signs of a developing eating disorder? How was I to know that her denial of hunger, avoidance of all situations that involved food, restricted and ritualistic eating habits, and excuses for not eating were symptomatic and that her anorexia had returned? How was I to know that Anna's decision to go on a diet when she was only 15 years old would prove to be fatal?

I did not have the information that could have helped me understand Anna's behaviors, thoughts, and feelings. When I was a young mom, nobody warned me that when I made comments about my size it could contribute to my young daughter questioning her size and shape. At that time I knew very little about anorexia, much less what to watch out for or how to help Anna if she developed the disease. When Anna was first diagnosed, there were few resources for family members, and accurate up-to-date information was hard to find.

As I read *100 Questions and Answers About Anorexia Nervosa,* I kept saying to myself "if only." If only this book had been available to me, Anna, and our family when we needed it, maybe things would have been different. If only I had known that Anna was vulnerable to developing an eating disorder because of her genetic makeup, her personality traits, and the culture she grew up in, I may have been able to intervene before she developed a full-blown eating disorder. If only someone had told me that puberty, life changes, and stressors could lead my daughter into an eating disorder. And finally, if only someone had told me that "dieting can be dangerous and can trigger behaviors and attitudes about weight that may progress into a more serious eating disturbance." If only *100 Questions and Answers About Anorexia Nervosa* had been available, maybe I would not have had to ask the one question that is almost unbearable: "How do you plan a funeral for a 21-year-old?"

Of course, we all know that hindsight is 20/20. Had I known then what I know now, I would have approached Anna's illness differently. After Anna died, I knew I had to use my experience to help others. Since her death in February 2000, I have talked with hundreds of family members of individuals suffering from anorexia, offering support and trying to answer some of the multitudes of questions they have. I have done countless interviews in an attempt to educate the public about eating disorders, and I have lobbied and testified before Congress to pass legislation that will improve access to care, allocate money for research, and develop education/prevention programs in our schools and communities.

When I began my work over 8 years ago, I felt like I was on my own trying to find answers for family and friends that would be meaningful and practical. It was not always easy or even possible to find the resources, and it could take hours of research to find what I thought was an answer based in research and sound clinical practice. The last thing I wanted was to give false and/or confusing information. *100 Questions and Answers About Anorexia Nervosa* is full of good information. It is practical and easy-to-read, and it answers many of the most frequently asked questions in an understandable, non-judgmental, and straightforward way. It should be on the bookshelf of every high school and public library in the country; it should be made available to all clinicians, educators, and community members who work with youth. Parents and loved ones should be given a copy when they are just beginning the journey into recovery from anorexia.

When my journey began over 13 years ago, I felt alone and very frightened and did not know where to turn. Today, I am happy to report, there is much more information available for family members, and Dr. Sari Shepphird's new book, *100 Questions and Answers About Anorexia Nervosa*, is a welcome addition to the growing list of resources for people who struggle with eating disorders, their family, and their friends. Thank you, Dr. Shepphird!

Kitty Westin
Founder, Anna Westin Foundation
(now the Emily Program Foundation)
President, Eating Disorders Coalition for Research, Policy & Action

Perhaps no mental illness is as misunderstood as anorexia nervosa. Misconceptions about the condition abound. For example, people may wonder: Is it a disease or a choice? Are people with anorexia merely trying to get attention, or is it a serious condition? Is it a "new" illness, or is the illness simply receiving more publicity of late?

100 Questions and Answers About Anorexia Nervosa is an effort to provide accurate, helpful information about this much-misunderstood illness. It was designed to assist patients, families, and other interested parties in obtaining important information about anorexia nervosa and to explain the illness's background, causes, warning signs, complications, and consequences. Related issues, such as body image and nutrition, are also addressed. Of course, a substantial part of this book discusses treatment as well as support for loved ones of anorexia patients. In addition, throughout the book, and in a separate Resources section at the end, I cite various organizations, printed materials, and Web sites that can further assist readers in their search for understanding. After all, 100 questions and answers are a great way to begin; however, I recognize that one book alone cannot contain all of the information that exists about this complex illness. Please take advantage of the resources provided, as each can offer further assistance in receiving much needed help and support.

This book is organized in parts, each part containing a number of questions and answers about the various aspects of anorexia nervosa. You will find a list of these parts in the Table of Contents. You may choose to read a specific part first, using the Table of Contents as a quick reference to a set of questions or for refreshing your memory about a particular subtopic. For a narrower search, you may wish to use the book's Index. Or, of course, you may read the book in its entirety. In addition to a listing of helpful resources, the back of this book also contains a glossary that explains some of the more technical terms you may encounter. You will also find these terms highlighted in **bold print** as you read, signaling that a definition is included nearby in the margin.

A note about my writing style and use of language: In speaking to patients and families throughout my nearly 20 years of exposure to anorexia nervosa, I have found that most are seeking straightforward, helpful answers to their important concerns and questions. You will find I try to be no less direct and straightforward in my writing. In my directness, you will notice I often shorten the term "anorexia nervosa" to simply "anorexia." This abbreviation occurs frequently in professional practice, thus I do so here as well. Sometimes, I use the terms "anorexia" and "eating disorder" interchangeably, as anorexia is one form of a broader category of eating disorders. I do this only when applicable and appropriate, but I make it known here for the sake of clarity. I also may occasionally use the terms "patient" and "client" interchangeably, a practice that frequently occurs within the healthcare community. With regard to word choice: When referring to individuals, I deliberately use the admittedly cumbersome phrases "he or she" and "his or her," rather than referencing a particular gender. It may make for some lengthy sentences, however, I prefer this to continuing the trend of exclusively identifying anorexia patients as "she." Although the vast majority of anorexia patients are indeed female, the illness has too long been stereotyped as a "female disease." Finally, I made a personal choice a long time ago not to use the term "anorexic" in referring to a person with the illness. Instead, I prefer the terms "anorexia patient" or "person with anorexia." Anorexia is an illness, separate from those who suffer from it. It is not one's identity, as the term "anorexic" may incorrectly imply.

ACKNOWLEDGMENTS

I would like to express my heartfelt gratitude to the many people who helped this project come to fruition. Among them, I would like to thank Ava Albrecht, MD, for her initial support and inspiration, as well as for her invaluable helpfulness along the way. I wish to thank Christopher Davis for providing me with this opportunity, and I would like to thank him, Jessica Acox, and Laura Almozara for their patience, understanding, and assistance. I wish to thank Kitty Westin for her contribution to this project and for her tireless efforts on behalf of patients and families who are affected by anorexia nervosa. My deepest appreciation goes to Lynn Bjorklund and Sarah Whitworth for contributing their insights and the wisdom of their experiences throughout the pages of this book. I offer my gratitude to Edward Tyson, MD, for his helpful suggestions. I also wish to genuinely thank those friends and colleagues who read the manuscript and offered practical feedback, and I extend my warm gratitude for the support and encouragement of those friends who not only helped me to stay focused, but also provided valuable distractions when needed! My love and appreciation also goes to my family, who has always conveyed confidence in me. Finally, I would like to thank my husband for his love and support, which mean more to me than words can express.

I wish there were no need for books about anorexia nervosa. Indeed, I wish anorexia and other eating disorders were not a threat to the lives and livelihood of countless girls and boys, women and men. I wish the young girls and boys who believe they are not "good enough" because they do not have the "perfect" body would see themselves as they really are—beautiful, irrespective of their weight or body type. I wish millions of families did not have to go through the pain and anguish of witnessing a loved one suffer from this illness. I wish those who exercise to the point of exhaustion would find rest from the compulsion that drives them to rid their bodies of unwanted calories. I wish no one would ever again encounter the belief that being thin is more important than being healthy. I wish a person at the brink of starvation would never again utter the phrase "you can never be too thin." I wish anorexia nervosa would not damage even one more body or mind. I wish no one—*not even one more malnourished individual*—would feel guilty for eating.

I wish anorexia nervosa were no more.

That is my wish list, a list shared by countless patients, former patients, families, and loved ones who have been confronted with the reality of this devastating illness.

Anorexia nervosa is a severe illness that daily threatens the health and well-being of those affected by it. It threatens to confuse and confound families even as it deprives its sufferers of a healthy body and mind. Although we are still a long way from seeing our wishes fulfilled, researchers continue to investigate the causes of this devastating illness, educators strive to increase understanding about anorexia in their communities, and healthcare providers work to enhance effective treatments for the disorder. This book is intended to be one small contribution toward the continuing effort of providing hope to patients, families, loved ones, and others who are seeking answers to the questions that comprise their individual "wish lists"—the wish of recovery, the wish of living a healthy and balanced life, the wish of finding support in the midst of great trial, the wish of sparing a loved one on the brink of anorexia the pain of this illness, the wish of feeling better equipped to share about anorexia with someone they love.

My hope is that patients and loved ones can find support and answers to the many questions they face. My hope is that interested professionals might feel better equipped to understand the illness and share that understanding with others. In fact *hope* is my purpose for writing this book. It is in that same hope that I long for the day when my "wish list" about anorexia nervosa will indeed become a reality.

Sari Fine Shepphird, PhD
Los Angeles, California

Lynn Bjorklund

I had my experience with anorexia as a teenager in the 1970s, when awareness of eating disorders was just beginning. I was a distance runner and fell into the trap of believing the "thinner the better." Weight loss and extreme training became obsessive, and my progression into anorexia and eating disorders put an end to my competitive running just at the time when I should have been at my best. Prior to that untimely ending, I managed to win several national cross country championships, competed with the U.S. international team in Russia, set an age group record for the 3000m, and set a long-standing record in the Pike's Peak Marathon. This demonstrates that an athlete with anorexia can do remarkably well for a period of time but still be headed for serious trouble. Resources for eating disorders back then were limited, so obtaining help wasn't always possible, which made for a very difficult struggle in achieving recovery. I am a great advocate now of prevention, early intervention, and the benefits of the great treatment opportunities that are available today.

Sarah Whitworth

Sarah Whitworth, 20, is a junior journalism major at the University of North Carolina (UNC) at Chapel Hill. Born and raised in Austin, Texas, Sarah evidenced some of the personality traits often seen in those with eating disorders. She placed high expectations on herself and strived to be the best at everything she did. With excellent grades, a blooming social life, and intensive training at a competitive dance studio, she appeared on the outside to be happy and healthy.

In eighth grade, Sarah decided she wanted to diet in order to lose three unwanted pounds and began restricting her food intake. After she lost the few pounds, she found herself caught in the dangerous and deadly cycle of what she would later come to realize was an eating disorder. She was diagnosed with obsessive-compulsive disorder (OCD) and anorexia nervosa her freshman year in high school. For four years, her life spiraled downward as she fell deeper and deeper into the depths of the anorexia.

After unsuccessful attempts at outpatient treatment, her family placed Sarah in the care of an inpatient treatment facility in 2004. The time she spent in the treatment center turned her life around; today she is physically and mentally healthier than ever. "I look at where I was in the depths of anorexia and where I am now," she says, "and know that I will never go back to that place with anorexia again."

Sarah is currently enjoying her journalism studies at UNC and is pursuing minors in Spanish and economics. Although she doesn't know what she wants to do with her life after college, one thing's for sure—it won't include battling an eating disorder.

PART ONE

Overview of Anorexia Nervosa

What is anorexia nervosa?

How is the diagnosis of anorexia determined?

Does anorexia only occur among teenagers?

More . . .

1. What is anorexia nervosa?

Psychiatric disorder

A recognized, diagnosable illness that results in the impairment of a person's cognitive abilities, emotional health, or interpersonal relationships; also called mental illness.

Anorexia nervosa, or "anorexia," is a serious and complex **psychiatric disorder** (also referred to as mental illness). Its symptoms include a severe disturbance in eating behavior, the inability or refusal to maintain a healthy body weight, and an intense fear of gaining weight. Disordered eating behaviors associated with anorexia include unhealthy weight loss and weight control methods (such as severe calorie restriction, food avoidance, or self-starvation) as well as inappropriate compensatory behaviors (such as excessive exercise, self-induced vomiting, or laxative abuse). Distorted self-perception of body shape and size is another hallmark of anorexia. Namely, people with anorexia may believe they are overweight and perceive themselves as fat even when they are underweight and extremely thin.

As with many other forms of mental illness, the symptoms associated with anorexia can be both confusing and frightening. Indeed, the consequences of the illness can be extremely dangerous and even deadly. Anorexia nervosa can have devastating effects on a person's physical, psychological, and social well-being. Yet for patients and their loved ones, gaining an understanding of the illness is the first step toward hope, healing, and recovery. Recovery from anorexia is possible and healing is attainable. The information in these pages will help.

Lynn shares:

I had anorexia for several years without ever realizing it. It is a disorder characterized by a lot of denial. I never realized that how I felt or behaved was anything other than what was necessary to be a fit and competitive athlete. The circumstances and manifestations leading to a diagnosis are varied, but it can be most surprising to finally realize one day that you are in the grip of a very dangerous disorder. I look back now and see that if I could have understood more about anorexia and what was happening, I might have recovered much more quickly and lessened the resulting consequences.

Breaking through that denial early on is very hard, but if success-ful, you can save yourself much further grief down the road.

2. How is the diagnosis of anorexia determined?

In many areas of medicine and healthcare, a diagnosis is made with the use of a diagnostic test, such as an x-ray or an MRI. In the case of psychiatric illnesses, however, a diagnosis is of-ten made on the basis of a patient's subjective report about his or her symptoms, sometimes along with a family's observation of the problem. There are medical tests that can measure the extent of physical complications of anorexia, but there is not a physical "anorexia test," per se. Instead, a diagnosis of anorexia nervosa, or any **eating disorder** for that matter, is made when a person's **symptoms** meet the diagnostic criteria given in the *Diagnostic and Statistical Manual of Mental Disorders*, 4th Edition (Text Revision), or **DSM-IV-TR** for short. Published by the American Psychiatric Association, the *DSM-IV-TR* provides a description of signs, symptoms, research findings, and guidelines that enable healthcare professionals to clas-sify mental illnesses. Appropriately trained mental health professionals use the *DSM-IV-TR* in order to determine the best descriptive category for a person's condition or problem. Before receiving a diagnosis of anorexia, a person receives a thorough professional assessment and a medical exam in order to rule out any physical conditions or illnesses that may be causing symptoms similar to those seen in anorexia nervosa.

The following are the diagnostic criteria for anorexia nervosa as they appear in the *DSM-IV-TR*, followed by a few clarify-ing phrases:

A. Refusal to maintain body weight at or above a mini-mally normal weight range for age and height (e.g., weight loss leading to maintenance of body weight less than 85% of that expected; or failure to make expected weight gain during period of growth, leading to body

Eating disorder

A severe disturbance in eating behaviors that results in an altered consumption of food and may significantly impair physical or mental health. An eating disorder is not diagnosed when the disturbed eating behaviors are the direct result of a general medical condition.

Symptom

A sign or indication of a disorder, disease, or condition.

DSM-IV-TR

A manual that qualified mental health professionals use to diagnose mental illnesses.

weight less than 85% of that expected). *This means that, according to the DSM-IV-TR, a person diagnosed with anorexia weighs roughly 85% or less of their ideal body weight as determined by standardized weight charts (or calculations of body mass) based on gender, height, and age. Most anorexia patients are of a normal weight when their symptoms first appear, however,* **pre-pubertal** *patients may acquire symptoms while they are still physically developing and therefore fail to reach a normal weight.*

B. Intense fear of gaining weight or becoming fat, even though underweight. *The type of fear referred to here is more intense than a typical person's concern about gaining a few pounds over the course of time.*

C. Disturbance in the way in which one's body weight or shape is experienced, undue influence of body weight or shape on self-evaluation, or denial of the seriousness of current low body weight. *Anorexia patients over-value their weight and appearance. Although anorexia patients may be able to accurately state if another person appears too thin, they tend to be inaccurate about the assessment of their own body shape and size. Even if emaciated, many people with anorexia deny that their condition merits serious concern.*

D. In **postmenarcheal** females, **amenorrhea**, i.e., the absence of at least three consecutive menstrual cycles. (A woman is considered to have amenorrhea if her periods occur only following hormone, e.g., estrogen, administration.) *Note: Many experts feel that this final criterion, amenorrhea, is too restrictive because some women who are at a very low weight continue to have their period, while some women lose their periods shortly after they begin dieting, even without extreme weight loss. Consensus suggests that patients with most of the key criteria of anorexia deserve to be diagnosed with this disorder and treated accordingly (Herzog and Eddy 2007). (See Question 7 for the male counterpart to the amenorrhea criterion.)*

In addition, the *DSM-IV-TR* specifies two *types* of anorexia nervosa (see Exhibit 1). When the diagnosis of anorexia

Pre-pubertal

Before the onset of puberty.

Postmenarcheal

Having established menstruation.

Amenorrhea

The absence of menstrual periods in females.

nervosa is given, a healthcare professional will also specify which type of anorexia best describes the associated pattern of behavior: *Restricting Type* or the *Binge-Eating/Purging Type*.

Exhibit 1   *DSM-IV-TR* Subtypes of Anorexia Nervosa

Restricting Type: during the current episode of anorexia nervosa, the person has not regularly engaged in binge-eating or purging behavior (i.e., self-induced vomiting, misuse of laxatives, diuretics, or enemas)

Binge-Eating/Purging Type: during the current episode of anorexia nervosa, the person has regularly engaged in binge-eating (eating of a significantly large amount of food during a given period of time) or purging (self-induced vomiting, misuse of laxatives, diuretics, or enemas)

SOURCE: American Psychiatric Association. (1994). *Diagnostic and statistical manual of mental disorders*, 4th ed., Text Revision (p. 589). Washington, DC: Author.

There is a second resource that may be used in diagnosing anorexia: the *International Classification of Diseases*, 10th Revision (*ICD-10*). Like the *DSM-IV-TR*, the *ICD-10* is a coding of signs, symptoms, and clinical findings that a healthcare professional might use to classify diseases and other health problems. Broader than the *DSM-IV-TR*, it is used internationally to classify all diseases and other health problems, including mental illness. A physician or other healthcare professional might utilize the *ICD-10* either in addition to or in lieu of the *DSM-IV-TR*. The descriptions of anorexia are similar in both references.

3. My doctor said I have "atypical anorexia." What does that mean?

Recall from the previous question that a diagnosis of anorexia requires that a person's symptoms meet a number of specific diagnostic criteria, as specified in the *DSM-IV-TR*. However, what happens when someone has symptoms of an eating disorder that do not meet all of these criteria? This occurs more frequently than you might imagine. Nancy Kolodny,

---

Exhibit 2 *ICD-10* Classification of Atypical Anorexia

Disorders that fulfill some of the features of anorexia nervosa but in which the overall clinical picture does not justify that diagnosis. For instance, one of the key symptoms, such as amenorrhea or marked dread of being fat, may be absent in the presence of marked weight loss and weight-reducing behavior. This diagnosis should not be made in the presence of known physical disorders associated with weight loss.

SOURCE: World Health Organization. (2007). *The international classification of diseases and related health problems*, 10th Rev. (Electronic Version). Retrieved July 22, 2008 from ICD-10 Online: www.who.int/classifications/apps/icd/icd10online

---

Bulimia nervosa

An eating disorder characterized by recurrent episodes of binge eating followed by inappropriate compensatory behavior, such as vomiting, misuse of laxatives, diuretics, enemas, or other medications; and/or fasting or excessive exercise. There are two subtypes of bulimia nervosa: purging type and non-purging type.

EDNOS

A diagnostic classification for several varieties of eating disorder symptoms classified in the *DSM-IV-TR*.

clinical social worker and author of *The Beginner's Guide to Eating Disorders Recovery*, states that as many as 10–20% of adolescent girls and young women display some, but not all, of the clinical symptoms of anorexia. Indeed, research findings indicate that *at least half* of all people diagnosed with an eating disorder do not meet the full criteria for either of the two primary eating disorders: anorexia nervosa and **bulimia nervosa**. In such cases, an alternative diagnosis is given. According to the *DSM-IV-TR*, "eating disorder not otherwise specified" (**EDNOS**) is the diagnostic term used to describe clinically significant eating disturbances that meet some, but not all, of the diagnostic criteria of either anorexia nervosa or bulimia nervosa. In the *ICD-10*, the corresponding term used is "atypical anorexia" (see Exhibit 2). Some of those diagnosed with EDNOS may have symptoms that closely align with diagnostic criteria of anorexia but fall outside of this diagnosis based on just one criterion. The differences between the diagnoses of anorexia and EDNOS are often a matter of fluctuating body weight and symptom severity. Indeed, a 2007 study showed that up to 70% of those diagnosed with EDNOS moved to a diagnosis of either anorexia or bulimia over a 30-month period. Therefore, it is important to note that a diagnosis of EDNOS is no less clinically significant than that of anorexia, nor is it necessarily of less concern. EDNOS can be quite serious and requires the same attention and level of treatment as another eating disorder diagnosis.

Examples of instances when a diagnosis of EDNOS (or atypical anorexia) might be given include:

- An individual who formerly met the diagnosis for anorexia nervosa returns to a normal weight, yet retains some, but not all, of the associated symptoms.
- An individual who does not express a fear of gaining weight, but nevertheless displays other symptoms of anorexia nervosa, including food restriction, weight-reducing behaviors, and substantial weight loss that is not due to any known physical illness.
- An individual of normal body weight who regularly uses inappropriate compensatory behavior (such as vomiting) after eating small amounts of food (two cookies, for example).
- An individual who repeatedly chews and spits out, but does not swallow, large amounts of food.

Perhaps case examples will serve as helpful illustrations. Let's begin with Barbara:

Barbara is a 5' 3", 26-year-old, recently married, Caucasian woman. Up until a month before her wedding day, Barbara weighed between 120 and 125 pounds, but she wanted to lose a few pounds before that day, thinking she would feel more comfortable wearing a bathing suit during her Hawaiian honeymoon. Barbara ended up losing a few pounds more than she planned, yet she liked the fact that her clothes fit a bit more loosely. Her husband made several comments about how much he liked her body when on their honeymoon, remarking that she was not "chunky," like his ex-girlfriend. When they returned from their honeymoon, several of Barbara's friends made comments about how "great" she looked. In fact, it seemed like the more weight she lost, the more her husband and acquaintances complemented her appearance. After losing 15 additional pounds, Barbara's mother grew concerned and told Barbara that she was "thin enough," yet Barbara did not change her diet. Instead, she became terrified that if she put any weight back on, her husband would no longer find her attractive. His verbal reassurances did not convince her otherwise.

By the time Barbara came in for treatment, she weighed 89 pounds. Barbara had severe, self-imposed food restrictions and stated that if she varied from these rules about food it made her feel "nervous for days afterward."

Barbara has a serious eating disorder. However, although her symptoms met *most* of the diagnostic criteria for anorexia nervosa, she was still having regular menses and therefore did not meet *all* of the diagnostic criteria for the disorder. Thus, Barbara was diagnosed with EDNOS.

Here is another case example:

Marc, an avid swimmer, is a 16-year-old Caucasian male with a history of childhood obesity. During the summer between his freshman and sophomore year of high school, Marc got a job as a construction assistant. He spent many hours carrying heavy loads of lumber, moving large bags of concrete, and climbing multiple flights of stairs. All of this activity left Marc 30 pounds lighter than when the summer began. Marc liked his new, slimmer appearance and vowed to maintain his weight loss after his summer job ended, but the methods he chose were not healthy. Marc severely restricted his calorie intake for days at a time and would frequently exercise to the point of exhaustion. Altogether, Marc lost about 20% of his body weight. In addition, he grew increasingly preoccupied with his weight and developed an intense fear of gaining weight.

Marc's symptoms are part of the diagnostic criteria for anorexia nervosa. However, Marc's current weight was still within the normal range. Therefore, his clinical presentation did not meet the full diagnostic requirements specified for anorexia nervosa. Instead, Marc's diagnosis was EDNOS.

4. I thought that when people make themselves vomit in order to lose weight, they have bulimia nervosa and not anorexia. Is this correct?

Actually, this is a common misconception. Let me help clarify the distinction between anorexia and bulimia, as they are currently defined within the *DSM-IV-TR*. The behaviors associated with anorexia and bulimia are often similar; the distinguishing factor between the two illnesses is the extent of weight loss in a patient. The diagnosis of anorexia only applies to an underweight patient. For example, a person engaging in binge eating or purging who weighs *less than* 85% of their expected normal weight would meet the diagnostic criteria for anorexia nervosa, while a normal-weight person who engages in similar behavior would be diagnosed with bulimia nervosa. As many as 40–60% of people who seek treatment for anorexia may engage in binge/purge behavior, so while these behaviors are commonly thought to be exclusive to bulimia, they are actually fairly common in anorexia as well (Hsu 1988). In fact, a person may be diagnosed with anorexia nervosa when he or she is severely underweight but receive a diagnosis of bulimia nervosa if the symptoms persist after weight-gain. Research has shown that approximately 20–50% of patients diagnosed with anorexia will at some time be diagnosed with bulimia nervosa, while nearly 25–30% of those with bulimia nervosa have a history of anorexia. Again, the key distinguishing factor is how much weight loss has occurred.

As many as 40–60% of people who seek treatment for anorexia may engage in binge/purge behavior.

5. What are the prevalence rates of anorexia nervosa?

For several reasons, precise numbers are difficult to attain. First, it is difficult to know with certainty the number of people affected by anorexia because, unfortunately, many who struggle with this condition do not seek help. Therefore, the information provided by **epidemiologists** reflects only the number of cases of anorexia actually seen in treatment. In

Epidemiologist

A person who studies the presence of disease in a population.

addition, reported prevalence rates tend to underestimate the total number of cases of anorexia due to the fact that many patients exhibit *some* of the symptoms of anorexia, but do not meet the full diagnostic criteria for the condition (see Question 2). Indications are, however, that anorexia is a rare but serious eating disorder that appears to be increasing in prevalence over time.

Anorexia ranks as the third most common chronic illness among adolescents, following obesity and asthma.

Scientific studies estimate that approximately 1% of the general population will develop anorexia at some point in their lives, and at least one of every 200 people will receive a clinical diagnosis of anorexia. We know that anorexia is less common than other eating disorders (such as bulimia nervosa and binge eating disorder) and that it is significantly less common than other forms of mental illness (such as depression and attention-deficit disorder). Nonetheless, anorexia ranks as the third most common chronic illness among adolescents, following obesity and asthma. Prevalence rates are the highest among adolescent girls and young women. According to the National Institute of Mental Health, approximately 0.5–3.7% of females will be diagnosed with anorexia nervosa in their lifetime. However, **partial-syndrome anorexia** is far more common. Researchers report that close to 5% of adolescent girls have this "mild form" of anorexia nervosa, displaying some, but not all, of the clinical symptoms of the disorder.

Partial-syndrome anorexia

A pattern of disordered eating in which a patient reports symptoms such as marked dietary restriction, weight preoccupation, and purging, but which fail to meet all of the diagnostic criteria for anorexia nervosa.

Incidence

The number of new cases of a disease in a defined population within a specified period of time.

Numerous reports indicate that **incidence** of anorexia has dramatically increased in the last few decades. Indeed, studies both in the United States as well as abroad seem to point to an increase in every decade since the 1960s. It is difficult to know for sure, however, whether the increase in rates of anorexia is the result of more accurate diagnostic methods, improved record keeping over time, an increased willingness of people to seek treatment, or an actual increase in the number of people with the illness.

One landmark review of medical records, published in 1991 by the *American Journal of Psychiatry*, would seem to confirm an actual rise in the rate of the condition. The chief researcher conducting this review, Dr. Alexander Lucas, utilized medical records that spanned a 50-year period (1935 to 1985) from the renowned Mayo Clinic, as well as those of the surrounding community of Rochester, Minnesota. He found that on average, the incidence rate increased by 35% for every 5-year period beginning in 1950 and ending in 1984. For those of us who work in the eating disorders field, and certainly for those whose lives have been affected by this disorder, this is indeed an alarming trend and a matter of great concern.

6. What is the history of anorexia nervosa?

The Encyclopedia of Obesity and Eating Disorders records that Simone Porta of Genoa, Italy, wrote the first medical account of anorexia in 1500. However, several hundred years would pass before the literature would offer detailed descriptions of the illness. Sir Richard Morton, a British physician, is credited with the first English-language description of anorexia in 1689. He reported of two adolescent cases, one female and one male, which he described as occurrences of "nervous consumption," a wasting away due to emotional turmoil.

In 1874, anorexia nervosa was introduced as a clinical diagnosis by two different physicians, Sir William Gull, of England, and Charles Lasègue, of France. Each emphasized varying aspects of the condition in their clinical reports, yet they both described anorexia as a "nervous" disease characterized by self-starvation. They were the first to recognize the illness as a distinct clinical diagnosis. When Gull reported about his work to the Clinical Society of London, he used the term *anorexia nervosa*, which literally means "nervous loss of appetite," to describe the condition. He was the first to do so. Gull's reports were published by the Society the following year, and the term later gained broad acceptance. Several prominent physicians of the nineteenth century described anorexia as a psychological condition, typically considered a form of hysteria or mental depression. However, it was not until the 1930s that physicians began to emphasize, for the first time, the value of psychotherapy in treating anorexia.

It is not as though extreme measures of weight control are new to the last few centuries of history. Accounts of self-starvation have been described at various points in the historical record. According to *The Encyclopedia of Obesity and Eating Disorders,* the ancient Greeks and Romans of the Classical period frowned upon obesity. Women of the upper social classes fasted in order to appear slim. Young people in ancient Sparta were said to have been examined in the nude monthly, and those who had gained weight were forced to exercise. According to Joan Jacobs Brumberg, author of *Fasting Girls: The History of Anorexia Nervosa*, in medieval Europe it was considered a miracle for a woman to engage in prolonged fasting. Religious literature of this era contains the accounts of many saints, mostly women, who restricted their eating out of spiritual concern. Fasting was considered a godly pursuit, while being overweight was often considered sinful and equated with gluttony. Today, according to Brumberg, the modern person with anorexia strives for aesthetic perfection to achieve a physical ideal, rather than a spiritual beauty.

According to Richard A. Gordon, author of *Eating Disorders: Anatomy of a Social Epidemic*, a watershed period of understanding the illness came with the modern 1970s work of noted eating disorders specialist, Hilde Bruch. Bruch argued that anorexia centered on issues of body image as well as disturbances in psychological development. She also proposed a third influence: a deficient "sense of self," which she characterized as a personal "ineffectiveness" that contributes to a struggle for personal autonomy, competence, and control. Bruch went on to comment on the process of therapy, which she perceived as helping a patient discover a "genuine self." In later works, she emphasized the importance of recognizing, defining, and challenging "erroneous assumptions and attitudes" and correcting errors in thinking that contribute to the onset and maintenance of the illness. In this way, she contributed immensely to modern approaches of psychotherapy and treatment for anorexia. Additional modern influences in the understanding of anorexia nervosa are Arthur Crisp, who describes anorexia as an attempt to control fears associated with maturity into adulthood, and Gerald Russell, who emphasizes the fear of fatness as a central component to the condition (Silverman 1997; Vandereycken and van Deth 2001).

Anorexia has only been a household word for a few decades. In 1983, the news of Karen Carpenter's death by heart failure resulting from anorexia fueled national attention. Television dramas, such as *Fame*, and made-for-TV movies, such as *The Best Little Girl in the World*, gave viewers the chance to learn about the impact of the disease. It was around this time that the doors opened at the Renfrew Center, the nation's first residential treatment facility devoted exclusively to eating disorders. Since that time, numerous recognizable names have been associated with anorexia. In the past few decades, research has dramatically increased our knowledge of the physical effects of starvation as well as the psychological and social components of anorexia. Precise, effective treatments have emerged, although there is much more work yet to do.

7. Does anorexia occur in males as well? Are there any differences in symptoms between males and females?

Yes, in fact, anorexia has been reported in male patients dating back to the seventeenth century, when London physician Richard Morton reported the first two documented cases of anorexia in 1694. One of his patients was a 16-year-old male. However, due to the current-day disparity in prevalence between the genders, the illness is generally, although incorrectly, regarded as a "female disorder." This is unfortunate because males do indeed develop anorexia nervosa, albeit much less commonly than females. Approximately 10–15% of those diagnosed with anorexia are male; however, that number appears

Approximately 10–15% of those diagnosed with anorexia are male; however, that number appears to be on the rise.

to be on the rise. Indeed, one of the fastest growing anorexia patient populations of the past decade is adolescent boys. Eating disorder specialist Leigh Cohn, coauthor of *Making Weight: Men's Conflicts with Food, Weight, Shape and Appearance*, states that therapists are seeing 50% more men for evaluation and treatment of eating disorders than just 10 years ago.

While eating disorder professionals believe that anorexia is under-diagnosed in both genders, additional factors make this of particular concern for males. Of particular note is that the *DSM-IV-TR* diagnostic criteria for anorexia includes amenorrhea, which is, of course, a strictly female concern (the *ICD-10* does include a male gender counterpart criterion of abnormal **gonadotropin** functioning). This may be one reason why healthcare professionals are less accustomed to suspecting anorexia in their male patients. Regardless, the danger is that some doctors may overlook, ignore, or misdiagnose male patients with this disorder. Additionally, Cohn and other specialists suggest that some men with anorexia may be unaware that they have an eating disorder, viewing symptoms such as excessive exercise and body shape concerns as just "a guy thing."

Gonadotropin

A group of hormones that affect the growth and function of the sex glands.

Gender stereotyping (e.g., regarding anorexia nervosa as a "female" condition) may be the root of what causes some males to refrain from seeking treatment. When they do, they will unfortunately find that there are far fewer residential treatment programs available to men than to women. Some co-ed programs do offer specially designed treatment "tracks" that address uniquely male concerns, but there is a need for many more such programs. Consequently, males with anorexia often report feeling isolated in treatment support groups composed of predominantly female patients. Nevertheless, the course of treatment for males is similar to treatment for female patients and generally has the same rates of **efficacy**. We have been making strides in recent years toward improving the diagnosis and treatment of males with anorexia, and this is indeed promising.

Efficacy

The extent to which an intervention produces an effect or beneficial result.

Certain male subgroups appear to be at a higher risk for anorexia. Athletes whose weight is a factor in their performance are an especially vulnerable group. Wrestlers, jockeys, runners, gymnasts, and dancers have a higher reported rate of eating disorders than the general population, due in part to the belief that weight loss is a necessary requirement for peak athletic performance in their sports. A higher rate of anorexia has also been reported in homosexual and bisexual males, with incidence reports as high as 20%. Other studies, however, have found no relationship between homosexuality and eating disorders, so the association remains in question. Researchers also caution that there is nothing about homosexuality itself that increases the likelihood of developing an eating disorder. Instead, higher prevalence rates may be attributed to stereotypes of physical attractiveness within the gay community and to increased help-seeking behaviors among gay males.

Important differences in the literature do exist between male and female eating disorder patients. For example, the research shows that men are more likely to engage in excessive exercise and less likely to engage in self-induced vomiting, use laxatives, or take diet pills to achieve desired weight loss. Some studies suggest that males are more likely to have co-occurring substance abuse. Research also shows that males appear to develop anorexia, on average, at a later age than females. One suspected reason for this is the later onset of puberty in boys. However, some studies have found a higher ratio of male to female anorexia cases in pre-pubertal aged children (Jacobs and Isaacs 1986).

8. Does anorexia only occur among teenagers?

The majority of new cases of anorexia are diagnosed in adolescents and young adults, most commonly between the ages of 13 and 18. The illness appears to have two peak ages of onset, one at puberty and the other in late adolescence (see Exhibit 3). However, anorexia does affect people of all ages and has been reported in patients as young as 7 and as old

> **Exhibit 3   Reported Age at Onset of Anorexia Nervosa**
>
> - 86% report onset of anorexia by the age of 20
>
> - 10% report onset of anorexia at 10 years of age or younger
>
> - 33% report onset of anorexia between the ages of 11 and 15
>
> - 43% report onset of anorexia between the ages of 16 and 20
>
> SOURCE: : The National Association for Anorexia Nervosa and Associated Disorders. (2008). *Facts about eating disorders*. Retrieved March 2, 2007 from: www.anad.org/22385/index.html

as 80. Recent research, in fact, indicates that older patients are being seen in increasing numbers. According to Carol Tappen and Holly Grishkat, Directors of the Eating Disorders Institute of St. Louis Park, Minnesota, and the Renfrew Center, respectively, eating disorders treatment centers have seen a significant increase in the number of patients over age 30. Experts suggest that factors such as growing public awareness, social pressure to be thin, and an aging population of "image conscious" baby boomers have produced this shift in the eating disorders treatment landscape.

Sub-clinical

The stage of development of an illness before symptoms are observed; or the presentation of symptoms of an illness that do not meet the full diagnostic criteria of an illness or condition.

Precipitating event

A triggering event that precedes and/or contributes to the development of an illness.

Cases of anorexia that *begin* in midlife and later adulthood have traditionally been considered rare. More commonly, we find that an older person with anorexia has experienced symptoms for quite some time, often beginning in adolescence. Often these patients either were misdiagnosed or did not seek prior treatment. Others may have experienced long-term struggles with body image, or **sub-clinical** symptoms of an eating disorder, and later developed anorexia after a **precipitating event** in adulthood. Yet the Renfrew Center reports that in 2005 about 20% of their adult eating disorder patients said they were age 30 or older when they first encountered symptoms. These numbers reflect an historical shift that has been witnessed by eating disorder professionals in recent years. Indeed, the most current scientific literature suggests a vulnerability to developing eating disorders *throughout* the lifespan.

Challenges such as divorce, childbirth, widowhood, menopause, and other age-related changes are examples of later-life events that may represent an increased vulnerability for at-risk individuals. Additionally, eating disorder experts believe that chronic dieting may pose a particular risk for anorexia and other eating disorders in women as they age.

We also know that body dissatisfaction, one of the most consistent risk factors associated with dieting and eating disorders, appears to be relatively stable across the lifespan. Studies show that middle-aged and older adults express high levels of dissatisfaction with their bodies, just as younger people do. According to a 1997 survey in *Psychology Today*, weight gain tops the list of negative influences on body image for both men and women between 13 and 90 years of age. Of those surveyed, two-thirds of the women and one-third of the men said weight gain had the greatest detrimental effect on their self-image. Thankfully, many healthcare professionals are becoming more aware of the possibility that eating disorders can develop later in life, and a number of treatment facilities offer specially designed treatment tracks for older patients.

Special Considerations for Mature Adults

The following are some special considerations for older adults regarding symptoms of anorexia:

- Even a person without a history of an eating disorder can develop anorexia at a later age. Be careful not to dismiss symptoms in an older person.
- Healthcare professionals may be less likely to suspect an eating disorder in an older adult, especially if a person has been functional for most of his or her adult life. If you suspect that you or a loved one may have anorexia later in life, persist at finding help and treatment with a qualified eating disorders professional.
- Thorough health and medical assessments are important. Physical illnesses, such as cancer, diabetes,

Parkinson's disease, cardiovascular illness, and certain infections can result in weight loss; therefore, it is vital to obtain an accurate diagnosis.

- While complications of anorexia are similar in patients both young and old, older patients may be more vulnerable to these complications.
- It is important for a healthcare professional to consider and rule out loss of appetite due to other mental illnesses, such as depression and dementia. Such illnesses can also co-occur with anorexia.
- It may be important with an elderly patient to include the family in treatment, especially with a non-emancipated individual.

Special Considerations for Children

There are also unique and important considerations when you suspect anorexia nervosa in a younger child. Some things to keep in mind:

Pica

A disorder characterized by the persistent eating of non-nutritive substances, such as dirt, clay, paper, or chalk.

Rumination disorder

A disorder in which a person, usually a child, regurgitates partially digested food before rechewing the food or spitting it out.

- Other childhood disorders can have a similar presentation to an eating disorder, so accurate diagnosis is essential.
- Feeding Disorders in children are a serious concern. The three most common feeding disorders in children are **pica, rumination disorder,** and failure to thrive. Other feeding behaviors such as food refusal, spitting out of food, food-related tantrums, and "picky" eating can be early risk factors for developing anorexia later in life. Be sure to discuss any unusual feeding practices with your child's pediatrician.
- Children with weight concerns before the age of 14 and those who report a higher incidence of stress or behavioral problems at a young age may be at a higher risk for eating disorders.

9. Is anorexia dangerous? What are the risks associated with anorexia?

Yes. Anorexia can be very dangerous. Indeed, the most serious physical risk associated with the illness is death. In fact, anorexia has the highest premature death rate of any mental illness, with estimates of fatality occurring in 5–20% of cases (the **aggregate death rate** is estimated at 0.56% per year or 5.6% per decade). The *American Journal of Psychiatry* reported that for female anorexia patients between the ages 15–24, the fatality rate associated with the illness is twelve times higher than *all other causes* of death. In addition, the suicide rate for people with anorexia is reportedly up to 50 times higher than in the general population. Most often, the cause of death for someone with anorexia is either from the physical complications of starvation or from suicide, and studies show that the risk of death from anorexia increases the longer one has had the illness. In addition, co-occurring psychiatric conditions (such as depression), substance abuse, and a high frequency of binge–purge behavior have been associated with increased risk of fatality.

Numerous additional medical complications can occur in patients with anorexia, many of which are the result of malnutrition (see Figure 1). Many of these medical complications can be quite serious, though some can be reversed through proper medical treatment and nutritional rehabilitation. Physical recovery, just like psychological recovery, can take a substantial amount of time, so it is important to consult a physician as soon as a problem is suspected and to include a medical doctor in the recovery process. Including a doctor is particularly important because certain medical illnesses can mimic many of the symptoms of anorexia. With a thorough examination, your doctor will be able to rule out other medical causes of symptoms resulting from a different diagnosis or condition. In the following paragraphs, you will find descriptions of some of the medical complications associated with anorexia (also see Table 1 for a more complete list of potential hazards).

Anorexia has the highest premature death rate of any mental illness.

Aggregate death rate

Sum or total death rate over time.

Overview of Anorexia Nervosa

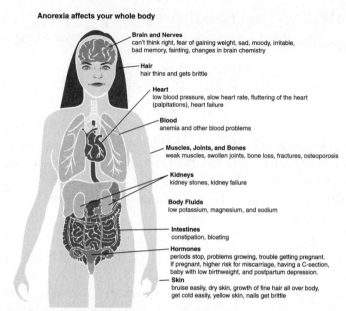

Anorexia affects your whole body

Brain and Nerves
can't think right, fear of gaining weight, sad, moody, irritable, bad memory, fainting, changes in brain chemistry

Hair
hair thins and gets brittle

Heart
low blood pressure, slow heart rate, fluttering of the heart (palpitations), heart failure

Blood
anemia and other blood problems

Muscles, Joints, and Bones
weak muscles, swollen joints, bone loss, fractures, osteoporosis

Kidneys
kidney stones, kidney failure

Body Fluids
low potassium, magnesium, and sodium

Intestines
constipation, bloating

Hormones
periods stop, problems growing, trouble getting pregnant. If pregnant, higher risk for miscarriage, having a C-section, baby with low birthweight, and postpartum depression.

Skin
bruise easily, dry skin, growth of fine hair all over body, get cold easily, yellow skin, nails get brittle

Figure 1   Organs and Systems of the Body Affected by Anorexia Nervosa
SOURCE: Office on Women's Health; U.S. Department of Health and Human Services.

Electrolytes

Salts that are found in the body, the most common of which are sodium, potassium, and chloride. A healthy balance of electrolytes is needed to maintain normal body function.

Arrhythmia

An abnormal or irregular rhythm of the heart.

Gastroparesis

Nerve or muscle damage in the stomach that causes slow digestion and gastric emptying, vomiting, nausea, or bloating.

Heart Problems

Self-starvation and the malnutrition caused by anorexia can have serious effects on one's heart and circulatory system. The malnourished heart muscle becomes weaker and may even shrink in size. Dehydration that results from purging or starvation can cause an imbalance of **electrolytes,** which may lead to an irregular heartbeat. In severe cases, cardiac **arrhythmia** can put a patient at greater risk for a heart attack.

Gastrointestinal Problems

Complications from anorexia can manifest in any part of the digestive system. Swollen glands, acid-reflux, and lesions in the esophagus can result from purging. Constipation is common with food restrictions. **Gastroparesis** can cause bloating, nausea, abdominal pain, and vomiting. The liver can develop deposits that may impair organ functioning. The use and abuse of laxatives can cause serious bowel perforations requiring surgical intervention (see Question 18).

Table 1   Medical Complications of Anorexia Nervosa

Organ System	Complications	Symptoms & Signs
Cardiac (heart)	Bradycardia (low heart-rate), decreased blood pressure, irregular heartbeat, heart murmurs, heart attacks, congestive heart failure, refeeding edema	Fatigue, weakness, dizziness, fainting, cold extremities, chest pain, shortness of breath
Gastrointestinal (digestive)	Obstipation, constipation, delayed gastric emptying, abnormal liver function, esophageal rupture, bowel perforations, internal bleeding, ulcers, gastritis, pancreatitis	Bloating, abdominal pain, vomiting, acid-reflux, heartburn, sore throat
Skeletal	Osteoporosis, arrested skeletal growth	Bone or joint pain with movement, delayed or suppressed growth, tooth loss
Brain	Organic Brain Syndrome, physical damage to the brain, brain shrinkage (decreased gray and white matter)	Cognitive difficulties, slowed processing, difficulty concentrating, forgetfulness, apathy, depression, increased risk of accidents and injury
Hematologic	Anemia, leukopenia (abnormally low number of white blood cells) with lymphocytosis, thrombocytopenia (low blood platelets), abnormal cytokines (proteins of the immune system)	Fatigue, cold intolerance, rare clotting abnormalities
Oropharyngeal (teeth and gums)	Dental decay, damage to gums, erythema in pharynx, enlarged salivary glands (effects due to purging)	Increased cavities, sensitive teeth, erosion of enamel, bleeding gums, swollen cheeks, sore throat and mouth, tooth loss, difficulty swallowing
Reproductive	Arrested maturation, fertility problems, serious pregnancy and perinatal complications, premature births	Amenorrhea, loss of libido, erectile dysfunction
Endocrine, metabolism	Hypothermia, dehydration, electrolyte imbalance, hypoglycemia	Low body temperature, fatigue, cold intolerance, vomiting, weakness
Skin and hair	Lanugo, Russell's Sign (scars on the hands), hypercarotenemia (skin discoloration), bruising easily	Fine hair or downy "fur" growth on skin and face, dry skin, brittle nails, calloused knuckles (from purging), hair loss or thinning, yellow skin

Overview of Anorexia Nervosa

21

Bone Problems

Anorexia can disrupt the regular bone growth of adolescents due to insufficient mineral availability resulting from a restricted diet. Boys and girls with anorexia are more likely to have growth deficiencies and are at heightened risk for severe bone disease as a result. Females, however, are especially susceptible to long-term bone problems. For example, **peak bone mass** is usually achieved prior to age 30. However, a young woman who develops anorexia as an adolescent may not reach peak bone mass, which places her at an increased risk for bone fractures and stunted growth. In addition, poor nutrition, low body weight, and decreased estrogen production resulting from malnourishment dramatically increase the likelihood of developing early **osteoporosis** in females. This higher risk is not just found in older women. Approximately half of young females with anorexia have osteoporosis, which can result in significant joint pain, tooth loss, bone fractures, and disability. In 2002, the *International Journal of Eating Disorders* reported that anorexia patients are twice as likely as those without anorexia to break a bone. This risk of bone fracture remains for 10 years after diagnosis.

It should also be noted that the results of recent research suggest that males with anorexia are likewise at increased risk for osteoporosis. Some of the potential consequences of osteoporosis and **osteopenia** are long lasting and may cause permanent skeletal damage. A **bone density test** can determine the extent of bone loss and can be used by physicians in determining if hormone replacement therapy, medication used for treating bone loss, or calcium supplementation may help restore bone density or prevent bone loss.

Lanugo

Lanugo is a fine, downy white hair that may grow on the body as a result of malnutrition. Referred to as "peach-fuzz," it is usually most noticeable on a patient's face, neck, arms, and back. Lanugo growth is one of the ways in which the body

Peak bone mass

The stage of growth at which bones have reached maximum density and strength.

Osteoporosis

A condition characterized by a progressive decrease in body density. Osteoporosis produces dry, brittle bones that may easily crack or collapse.

Approximately half of young females with anorexia have osteoporosis.

Osteopenia

A decrease in bone density that is less severe than in osteoporosis.

Bone density test

A test that measures the strength and density of bones; often used to determine the risk of developing osteoporosis. Also called bone mineral density (BMD) test.

Lanugo

A fine, downy white hair that may grow on the body as a result of malnutrition.

attempts to adjust to the slowing down of the metabolism that occurs with prolonged fasting and weight loss. With any significant weight loss that reaches the point of semi-starvation, the body's core temperature drops; patients in this state report feeling cold most of the time as a result. Lanugo is, in essence, a way that the body tries to keep itself warm. It is not, in itself, harmful, but signals that the body has reached dangerous levels of malnutrition. It does not grow in all cases of anorexia, but it can be frightening when it does occur. Lanugo can be reversible, and the key is to get one's body back to a healthy state where it is nourished and well-fed.

Lynn shares:

During my years in anorexia, I can remember running a race on a hot day and toward the end of it, having the sensation of my whole body cramping up. It felt like I was in one of those slow motion dreams. I finished the race (even won it), but later felt all sorts of heart arrhythmias that were very frightening. Much later, when I finally saw a doctor, blood work results showed one of the lowest blood potassium levels ever seen in an ambulatory patient. You can look quite normal, even perform superbly well, yet be in a very dangerous state.

I developed anorexia just before puberty. As a result I never started my periods until age 28. Throughout the eating disorder, powdered milk was a mainstay for me, and I was very active with weight bearing exercise. I theorized that this combination might save me from the predicted bone loss. Following recovery, and for the next two decades, I continued with everything possible to achieve and maintain good bone health—adequate calcium and associated vitamins and minerals, strength training, and weight bearing exercise. At age 50 I was still diagnosed with osteopenia of the spine.

10. Can you help me to understand the thoughts and feelings associated with my loved one's illness?

It can certainly be difficult for someone who has not experienced anorexia to understand the thoughts and feelings associated with the illness. While every person with an eating disorder is different and experiences their own unique set of emotional challenges, some common themes have been reported. The first of these themes may come as no surprise: People with anorexia think a great deal about food. In fact, most anorexia patients report that thoughts about food, weight-control, and body image are an all-encompassing preoccupation. "If I was not thinking about my food and weight, I don't know what else I would think about. It's all that I do all day," a patient recently confessed to me. It was not the first time someone had expressed this sentiment.

More than just counting calories, weighing oneself, and avoiding so-called "bad" foods, weight control can become a measuring stick for life and success. A "good" day is when one restricts eating to an acceptable degree; a "bad" day is when one has consumed more than their daily "allotment of calories." Likewise, some patients use body image as their compass. Thus, a "good" day is when clothes fit loosely and the stomach appears flat; a "bad" day is feeling bloated or having the stomach protrude. Personal identity and self-worth become intertwined with weight and appearance. Weight gain may be experienced as a personal failure with accompanying feelings of guilt and shame. In contrast, being the "thinnest one" in a room full of people may be experienced as virtue and victory. While it may indeed be hard to understand the extent to which anorexic thoughts preoccupy a patient's life, it may be helpful to learn of some associated patterns. Your loved one may:

- Count calories at every meal
- Plan what they will eat far in advance

- Be attentive to bodily sensations, such as feeling bloated or full
- Be overly concerned with other's evaluations of them
- Compare themselves to others
- Feel fat, even when they are not
- Use weight control as a measure of personal success or failure
- Experience compliments as reinforcements for their weight control efforts
- Divide foods into "good" and "bad" categories and rate themselves as "good" or "bad" if these foods are consumed
- Pursue perfection through weight control
- Be overly sensitive to remarks about personal appearance
- Deny their own need for food and nourishment
- Plan ways to purge food or compensate for food consumption (e.g., exercise)
- Experience persistent, incessant negative self-evaluation (e.g., "you're fat!" "you have no willpower!" "you're a failure!")

While this list is illustrative of the kinds of thoughts that preoccupy a person with anorexia, the ironic thing is that the issues that may underlie anorexia symptoms often have very *little* to do with food. In reality, the preoccupations associated with anorexia can sometimes serve as a distraction from, and a complex means of coping with, deeper psychological pain or turmoil. Take Jeanie, for example:

The issues that may underlie anorexia symptoms often have very little to do with food.

Jeanie is a 19-year-old gymnast who dreamed of competing at the highest levels of her sport. She began her training at age four and was considered a "natural" by her parents and coaches. Jeanie loved going to classes and later to training-practice, often showing her enthusiasm by dancing around the equipment in between routines, her favorite songs playing on the radio in the background.

Tragedy struck Jeanie's life when she was 11 years old. She and her family were bike riding on a familiar road near their home when an out-of-control driver struck the bike that her brother was riding and he was killed. Jeanie recalls the event as "the day that my light went out inside." Jeanie and her family were understandably distraught for many months. Her parents, however, continued to take Jeanie to practices and attend her meets without interruption. They felt it would not be fair to stop Jeanie from enjoying her gymnastics and admittedly found it "therapeutic" to cheer Jeanie on to do her best.

Jeanie began to feel the pressure of competing in a completely new way. It was no longer a fun way to spend her time. Instead, Jeanie threw herself deeper into training, not only for herself and her team, but also "in order to help me and my family heal." Jeanie thought that by becoming the best gymnast on the team, she could erase the pain she and her parents were experiencing. As Jeanie's body began to change with puberty, she became increasingly concerned about gaining weight. She says she felt pressure to "not let anything get out of balance" in her life, and her weight was one of those "things." Jeanie began restricting her food intake, yet all the while maintained a rigorous training schedule. Eventually, Jeanie was diagnosed with anorexia nervosa and admitted to the hospital for complications related to malnutrition.

As Jeanie's story illustrates, for some patients, anorexia symptoms provide an emotional anesthetic, numbing feelings and offering retreat into a "safe" world constructed by the illness.

Lynn shares:

I remember the feeling that no matter what I did, it was never good enough. I could get straight A's in school, but I considered myself stupid and unworthy. I could win a national championship in running, set a national age group record, win a prestigious race, but I still couldn't feel good about myself or like myself. I was greatly embarrassed by any recognition of my accomplishments, feeling like I really didn't deserve it. If I won a race or set a record, it was just a lucky moment in time or a sort of accident, and I would then try to do better next time. I was constantly and ravenously hungry, yet believed I didn't deserve to eat and was afraid to eat.

Even though it wasn't working, it seemed that striving to be a good athlete and being very thin might somehow relieve my extreme feeling of unworthiness and self hate. I imagined that anyone who met me would automatically dislike me as much as I did. It was a tortuously lonely existence, so I put all of my thoughts and efforts into being a good runner and being as thin as possible. These were synonymous for me; being a good runner and being as thin as possible. I didn't believe you could have one without the other. The resulting starvation and exhaustion often blocked the feelings of loneliness, self hate, and despair.

Sarah shares:

Anorexia was a horrible, life-consuming experience. Sometimes I still don't understand the thoughts and feelings I had during my illness. At any given time, I was calculating the number of calories I had taken in during the day and the amount I needed to run to cancel out these calories.

But as my doctor tells me to this day, "Anorexia is not about fat, food, or figure. It's about feelings." As much as I never believed him when I was in the midst of the disorder, he was right. I used anorexia as a mechanism to cover up feelings I didn't even know I had, to distract myself from bigger issues that were at hand in my life.

11. Do people with anorexia get better?

The good news is that for the majority of people with anorexia, the answer is *yes*! It takes time, support, and often a great deal of effort, but *recovery is possible*. Most studies suggest that the majority of people with anorexia achieve some degree of recovery (75–80%), although the length of treatment will vary for each individual. However, anorexia can be difficult to treat, and while most people do recover, not everyone does. Of those who seek treatment, about half recover completely, about 25–30% make significant progress, and about 20% have chronic symptoms of the illness. Yet studies indicate that even individuals with long-standing anorexia can show improvement. Outcomes are significantly better with early treatment, so seeking help early in the course of anorexia is always advised. Studies indicate that adolescents may recover more quickly than older adults, and patients who have been hospitalized have a better recovery outcome if they reach a normal weight prior to discharge. Some key factors that have been negatively associated with recovery are chronic low weight, the presence of certain coexisting psychiatric conditions, lack of support for treatment within a patient's family, and lack of follow-up treatment.

Lynn shares:

Recovery can be very hard and is often not a smooth or easy path. Even so, it is very much achievable, and the work, learning, and accomplishments in recovery benefit every aspect of your life. You can come out of recovery with the tools to meet life challenges in ways that you would never have had otherwise. The team of professionals often needed for that recovery process can be very expensive, but it will be the best investment, with the greatest returns, that you may ever make.

Sarah shares:

Recovering from anorexia was without a doubt the most difficult thing I have ever done in my life. But looking back at how far I have come since I received treatment in 2004, I know that I'll never go back to my eating disorder again. Depending on my stress level and other outside factors, it's not uncommon for eating disordered thoughts to enter my head; I've just learned to ignore them when they do come up. I think of it as the "Beautiful Mind" analogy: Even years after John Nash "recovered" from his schizophrenia and although he is a distinguished scholar who received the Nobel Prize, he stills sees the imaginary roommate and girl that were once his best friends. They are always there, but he has to realize that they are only in his imagination, and he learns to ignore them.

PART TWO

Weight Loss and Other Warning Signs

What is "starvation syndrome"?

Before my son developed anorexia, I thought it was only a problem for girls. What are some other myths about anorexia?

It seems like there are many reasons why a person might lose appetite and not eat for a period of time. How can one know if anorexia is the cause?

More . . .

12. I am concerned that my roommate may have anorexia, but I am not certain. Are there any behaviors or warning signs that I should be watching for?

A diagnosis of anorexia nervosa is established after a thorough examination by a healthcare professional. However, there are some behavioral signs, or "red flags," that may signal a reason to be concerned. Early intervention and treatment are shown to assist in the recovery from anorexia, so it is important to speak to loved ones and encourage talking to a healthcare professional as soon as you suspect a problem.

With gratitude to Anorexia Nervosa and Related Eating Disorders, Inc. (ANRED) and the Multiservice Eating Disorders Association (MEDA), the following checklists present warning signs associated with anorexia nervosa. The signs are grouped into different behavior categories for the sake of clarity. Someone with anorexia nervosa may exhibit some or all of these symptoms. Many of the signs and symptoms listed can also be signs of other illness, so be sure to consult a trained professional for a complete evaluation and proper diagnosis. In addition, Exhibit 4 contains a self-test that highlights many of the prominent symptoms of anorexia.

Food Behaviors

Circle behaviors observed:

- Denies hunger
- Will only eat a few "safe" foods
- Avoids eating with others
- Cooks for others but does not eat what is prepared
- Is ritualistic about food (e.g., chews each bite a certain number of times, measures food servings, counts the number of food items eaten) or has other rules about eating (e.g., will not eat past a certain time)
- Restricts eating or maintains severe dieting

Exhibit 4   Eating Disorders Self-Test

Do You Have an Eating Disorder?

Respond honestly to these questions. Do you:

- Constantly think about your food, weight, or body image?
- Have difficulty concentrating because of those thoughts?
- Worry about what your last meal is doing to your body?
- Experience guilt or shame about eating?
- Find it difficult to eat in public?
- Count calories whenever you eat or drink?
- Still feel fat when others tell you that you are thin?
- Obsess that your stomach, hips, thighs, or buttocks are too big?
- Weigh yourself several times daily?
- Feel that the number on your scale determines your mood and outlook for the day?
- Punish yourself with more exercise or restrictions if you don't like the number on the scale?
- Exercise more than an hour every day to burn calories?
- Exercise to lose weight even if you are ill or injured?
- Label foods as "good" and "bad"?
- Vomit after eating?
- Berate yourself if you eat a "forbidden" food and compensate by skipping your next meal?
- Use laxatives or diuretics to keep your weight down?
- Severely limit your food intake?

If you answered "yes" to any of these questions, regardless of whether you fit the diagnostic criteria for an eating disorder, your attitudes and behaviors about food and weight may need to be addressed. A professional familiar with the treatment of eating disorders can give you a thorough assessment, honest feedback, and advice about what you may want to do next. You may find it helpful to share your thoughts, concerns, and feelings with someone who can listen compassionately while suspending judgment. At the very least, you deserve help maintaining your physical and medical safety, something that an eating disorders professional can provide.

SOURCE: Adapted from Hall, L., and Ostroff, M. (1999). *Anorexia nervosa: A guide to recovery.* (pp. 29–30). Carlsbad, CA: Gürze Books. Used with permission.

- Purges (i.e., self-induced vomiting)
- Makes frequent trips to the bathroom after eating (can be a sign of purging)
- Hoards food
- Eats alone; eating patterns are vague or secretive
- Overuses caffeine
- Skips meals
- Chews food and spits it out before swallowing
- Makes excuses for not eating; plays with food on plate, or moves it around, instead of eating
- Is preoccupied with food content and ingredients
- Divides food into "good" and "bad" based on fat content
- Suffers intense guilt after eating

Appearance and Body Image Behaviors

- Has lost significant weight and/or refuses to maintain minimum normal weight
- Exhibits great concern about weight; shows intense fear of gaining weight; complains of "feeling fat"
- Spends time inspecting self in mirror
- Entertains magical thinking about weight (e.g., "If I am thinner, I will feel better about myself.")
- Seeks to emulate thin people
- Wears baggy clothes to hide weight loss
- Weighs self frequently
- Has negative body image
- Weight fluctuates
- Abuses diet pills or prescription medications

Exercise Behaviors

- Exercises even when injured or overly tired
- Exercises compulsively

Thoughts, Beliefs, and Feelings

- Difficulty expressing feelings that are not related to food or weight
- Suicidal thoughts
- Depression (may include feelings of shame, anger, or guilt)

- Self-critical and/or a "perfectionist"
- Overly concerned with opinions of others; may be described as a "people-pleaser"
- Extremes in thinking (e.g., "all or nothing thinking"; see Question 88)
- Low self-esteem, feelings of worthlessness
- Mood fluctuations, irritability
- Difficulty concentrating
- Isolated, withdrawn
- Impaired relationships

Physical Complaints

- Abdominal cramps, bloating
- Decreased coordination
- Headaches
- Dental problems, swollen glands, discolored teeth
- Hair loss
- Dry skin, bruises
- Bloodshot eyes
- Insomnia
- Constipation, gastrointestinal problems
- Frequent complaints about being cold
- Fatigue, or in contrast, hyperactivity
- Complaints of nausea
- Dizziness or fainting
- Growth of fine, downy body hair

Other Behaviors

- Self-mutilating behaviors (e.g., hitting, burning, or cutting oneself)
- Denial of symptoms
- Substance use or abuse
- Suicidal gestures
- Dramatic weight loss
- Frequent use of laxatives or diuretics

While all of these "other" behaviors can raise concern for anorexia, their appearance, even in isolation, is associated with an additional increased risk of harm. Professional attention is strongly recommended.

Sarah shares:

I used to constantly worry about what other people were eating and would compare my daily intake to that of my close friends. I meticulously planned out every little detail of when/where/what I ate, and rigidly stuck to my self-created rules. To anyone who spent a significant amount of time with me, it was pretty apparent that something wasn't right.

13. What is "starvation syndrome"?

Starvation syndrome refers to the psychological and physiological effects of starvation on a person's mind, body, and behavior. Many of the changes that take place in the thinking and behavior of a person with anorexia are due to the effects of starvation, or **semi-starvation**. An important research study from the 1950s has dramatically increased our understanding of the impact of restrictive dieting and weight loss on otherwise healthy individuals. Ancel Keys and his colleagues from the University of Minnesota conducted an experiment with 36 healthy young men who agreed to be monitored before, during, and after a period of severe, imposed dietary restrictions and resulting weight loss. During the dieting phase of the experiment, the men lost an average of 25% of their original weight. These men experienced dramatic changes, not just physically, but also in their psychological functioning and social behavior. A summary of these changes can be found in Exhibit 5 and includes food preoccupation, depression, anxiety, irritability, social withdrawal, decreased concentration, poor judgment, sleep disturbances, decreased sexual interest, apathy, and personality changes.

Keys and the other researchers noted that the men became intensely focused on thoughts about food; they dreamed about food, they read about food, and some men who showed no prior interest in cooking began collecting recipes and kitchen

Many of the changes that take place in the thinking and behavior of a person with anorexia are due to the effects of starvation.

Semi-starvation

The state of being partially or nearly starved.

Exhibit 5   Natural Results of Semi-Starvation

Attitudes and Behavior Toward Food	*Emotional and Social Changes*
Food preoccupation	Depression
Collecting recipes, cookbooks, menus	Anxiety
	Irritability
Unusual eating habits	Anger
Increased consumption of coffee, tea, spices	"Psychotic" episodes
	Personality changes
Gum chewing	Decreased self-esteem
Binge eating	Social withdrawal
Cognitive Changes	*Physical Changes*
Decreased concentration	Sleep disturbances
Poor judgment	Weakness
Apathy	Gastrointestinal disturbances
	Hypersensitivity to noise and light
	Edema (water retention)
	Hypothermia and feeling cold
	Decreased metabolic rate
	Decreased sexual interest
	Hair loss

SOURCE: Keys, Brozek, Henschel, Mickelsen, and Taylor. (1950). Adapted from Garner, D., and Garfinkel, P. (1997). *Handbook of treatment for eating disorders*. (p. 103). New York: The Guilford Press.

utensils. Irritability, depression, and outbursts of anger were seen in men who previously showed no signs of such dispositions prior to the experiment. Many of the men became socially withdrawn. Some who showed no prior body image dissatisfaction began to be more critical of their bodies and complained of being overweight. Others attempted to lose additional weight through deliberate exercise.

If you are thinking that the effects of starvation on the men in Keys' experiment sound similar to the symptoms displayed in anorexia, you are indeed correct. Psychologist David Garner writes in the *Handbook of Treatment for Eating Disorders*, "One of the most important advancements in the understanding of eating disorders is the recognition that severe and prolonged dietary restriction can lead to serious physical and psychological complications. Many of the symptoms once thought to be primary features of anorexia nervosa are actually symptoms of starvation."

The significance of this experiment cannot be understated. Even behavioral changes such as depression, anxiety, and feelings of guilt about weight and food can be understood as part of a natural human response to starvation. Keys' work also underscores the importance of normal weight restoration as an essential element in the recovery from anorexia.

14. When my doctor weighs me during checkups, she refers to my body mass index instead of my weight. What is the difference?

Body mass index (BMI) is a measurement used by physicians and eating disorders professionals as an indicator of total body fat. It does not measure body fat directly but has been found to correlate with other direct measures of body fat. It is used in conjunction with a thorough health screening and is often preferred over height/weight tables for determining a healthy weight range in adults. A person's BMI is calculated using the following formula:

$$\text{BMI} = \frac{\text{Weight (in pounds)}}{(\text{Height in inches})^2} \times 703$$

While individual variations do occur, the National Institutes of Health provides guidelines for a healthy BMI range (see Table 2). The ranges included apply to adults; the BMI measurement applies differently to children. With children, a BMI percentage for an individual child is compared to BMI measurements for children of the same age and gender. Generally, children with a BMI below the fifth percentile for age and gender are considered underweight. Readers can visit *www. cdc.gov* and click on "BMI Calculator" to calculate an adult's or child's BMI.

Table 2   Body Mass Index Guidelines

BMI	Weight Range
Below 18.5	Underweight
18.5–24.9	Normal
25.0–29.9	Overweight
30.0 and Above	Obese

Limitations of BMI

BMI is a calculation based on weight and height and cannot provide any additional detail about body composition (e.g., percentage of body fat). BMI measurements do not distinguish between body fat mass and lean tissue mass, nor do they consider one's frame size. Therefore, BMI calculations may be over-inflated in an athletic or very fit person due to a higher percentage of muscle mass. Likewise, a BMI calculation may not be as accurate for an elderly person with reduced bone density and muscle mass. Other factors such as ethnicity, pregnancy, adult age, gender, physical activity, and bone structure can produce variations in a BMI measurement.

15. What is the "set-point theory" of weight regulation?

Set-point is a concept that refers to a body's natural weight range that is "set" by factors such as heredity, health, age, gender, body frame, and level of physical activity. Similar terms used include "settling point," "natural weight," and "regular weight." These terms describe the weight range at which one's body is the healthiest and is usually maintained by eating a normal amount of food and engaging in a normal, healthy amount of physical activity. For children and adolescents, set point is part of a normal pattern of genetically predetermined growth and development. Every person has a unique set-point—not one number on the scale, but a *range* of weight that is within the body's own natural equilibrium.

As a helpful illustration, consider a thermostat. When a thermostat is set at a certain temperature, it will regulate heating and cooling systems in order to maintain the set temperature. Likewise, our bodies have a certain weight "temperature" to which they will naturally gravitate. This temperature is unique to each individual. Some people may tend to gravitate toward the lower range of their set point, others toward the higher end. Fluctuating within this healthy weight range is normal. The human body will tend to resist changes in weight that go beyond set-point range. Thus, practically speaking, if a person misses a meal during the day, the body responds with sensations of hunger in order to increase the desire to eat. Likewise, if a person loses weight below their set-point range, the body compensates by reducing its **metabolic rate** in an attempt to return itself to a normal weight. Experts believe that set-point theory may explain why food binges often follow a period of caloric restriction: The body is attempting to ingest the nutrients and energy that it needs in order to maintain a healthy equilibrium.

Metabolic rate

The rate of energy production in the body.

16. Before my son developed anorexia, I thought it was only a problem for girls. What are some other myths about anorexia?

That is a great question because the misconceptions about this illness abound. What follows are some frequently voiced myths and misconceptions about anorexia, followed by facts that refute each myth.*

People do not choose to have anorexia. Anorexia, like other forms of eating disorders, is a serious illness.

Myth: People choose to have anorexia.
Fact: People do not choose to have anorexia. Anorexia, like other forms of eating disorders, is a serious illness.

Myth: Eating disorders are primarily about food and weight.
Fact: Anorexia and other eating disorders are *not* solely a problem with food. Behaviors such as food restriction, fasting, and purging are *symptoms* of underlying issues.

---

* Portions of this information were adapted with permission from *Eating Disorders: The Journey to Recovery Workbook* and *Eating Disorders: Time for change* (Villapiano and Goodman 2001).

Myth: Individuals with anorexia are just trying to get attention.
Fact: People do not develop anorexia as a way to seek out attention. Although it is maladaptive, anorexia can sometimes serve as a person's way to cope with something painful in his or her life.

Myth: Anorexia is about vanity. If a person with anorexia says, "I feel fat," it is just to get compliments.
Fact: People with anorexia experience a real distortion in their body image. This is one of the symptoms of the illness. Often, a person with anorexia will view his or her body very differently than we view it. Described as looking in a "fun-house mirror," the self-perceptions of people with anorexia are not an accurate reflection of their true body weight and shape (see Question 43).

Myth: Anorexia is a rich, young, white girls' problem.
Fact: Research has shown that this is not true. A person with anorexia may be from any racial, ethnic, or economic background (see Question 29). Anorexia does not discriminate. It affects young and old, female and male.

Myth: People with anorexia do not engage in binge eating.
Fact: People with anorexia may sometimes engage in binge eating. Binge episodes are often followed by an attempt to purge what has been consumed through the use of laxatives, vomiting, or excessive exercise.

Myth: A person cannot have anorexia if they eat three meals a day.
Fact: Fasting is not the only means of food restriction. It may be that a person limits the *types* of food eaten or the *amount* of food eaten. For example, a person may eat a normal amount of food for several days and then follow this with severe calorie restriction. A related misconception is that people with anorexia do not eat junk food, only healthy food. This is not necessarily the case. In fact, people with anorexia may eat sugary foods in order to maintain their physical energy.

Myth: You cannot die from anorexia if you exercise to keep your heart and body strong.

Fact: People with anorexia may believe this myth in an attempt to convince themselves that their illness is not serious. Some believe that taking vitamin supplements will protect their bodies from the effects of malnutrition or that they will not face health risks if they avoid certain well-publicized eating disorder behaviors. Yet the medical complications of starvation and malnutrition are real.

Myth: If my loved one would just eat, she would be fine.

Fact: To be sure, returning to a normal weight is an important part of recovery from anorexia nervosa. However, just telling your loved one to eat more will not make anorexia go away. It is important that your loved one seek help for their eating disorder.

Myth: Someone is to blame for this eating disorder.

Fact: There are many different reasons why someone develops anorexia, and multiple risk factors have been identified (see Question 22). While trauma and other stressors can be a contributing factor, we now know that anorexia has a complex **etiology**. Fortunately, we are learning more and more about various biological, psychological, and sociological factors that contribute to the development of eating disorders. The more we know, the more we are able to provide effective treatment.

Myth: If I tell someone about my eating disorder, they will just try to make me fat.

Fact: Getting help is not about getting fat; it is about becoming healthy and getting your life back. It is common to feel nervous about beginning the recovery process, but do not let it keep you from getting help. Your doctor or therapist is not trying to take away your sense of control; they are trying to help empower you toward healing.

It is important that your loved one seek help for their eating disorder.

Etiology

The cause or origin of a disease, condition, or illness.

Myth: Anorexia is all about control.

Fact: There is some truth to this statement, but it is important to clear up any misconceptions surrounding the idea of control and eating disorders. A person with anorexia may feel that he or she has been unable to effect change in certain aspects of life or may feel unable to control the unfolding of certain life events. He or she may instead attempt to control food intake as a way of having mastery over one area of life. For some patients, anorexia serves as a complex distraction from other painful, seemingly unmanageable feelings or events. A person with an eating disorder does not know of another way to cope, but most would change this if they could. Part of the recovery process is acquiring other, healthier ways of coping with life's challenges.

Myth: Anorexia is just a "phase."

Fact: Anorexia is never normal behavior. It is an eating disorder that needs serious attention.

Myth: You can never recover from anorexia.

Fact: You *can* recover. Recovery can take time, but with the help of treatment, *it is possible.* It is important to seek help as soon as you suspect an eating disorder.

Myth: There is nothing I can do to make my loved one recover.

Fact: It is true that you cannot *make* your loved one recover. However, there are things that you can do to support your loved one's recovery (see Questions 50–60).

Lynn shares:

Another myth might be that "all people with anorexia eat very little, if any, food." The diagnosis of anorexia in my case was missed because it appeared that I ate normally and seemed to function and perform well. As a distance runner, I even ate more than most people my age, consuming at least 2500 to 3000 calories per day. Even so, my exercise level was so extreme that I continually lost weight. Most people thought I was a big eater, but I was constantly ravenous because I wasn't meeting my calorie needs, even with what might have looked like a lot of food. I was still deliberately restricting food intake so that I always remained in a negative calorie balance. I later learned how such intensive training and nutritional deprivation can be very dangerous.

17. It seems like there are many reasons why a person might lose appetite and not eat for a period of time. How can one know if anorexia is the cause?

Anorexia nervosa can both mimic and co-occur with physical illnesses that have similar symptoms.

Colitis

An inflammation of the large intestine (colon). Symptoms may include abdominal pain, fever, and severe diarrhea.

Addison's disease

A disease caused by a deficiency of hormones that are produced by the adrenal gland. Symptoms may include weight loss, fatigue, and vomiting.

Anorexia nervosa can both mimic and co-occur with physical illnesses that have similar symptoms, so it is important to have a thorough evaluation when an eating disorder is suspected to rule out the presence of other conditions. A first step would be to have a family physician, particularly one who is familiar with eating disorders, conduct a complete physical exam to determine if any of these conditions exist. Physical disorders that may display similar symptoms to anorexia include diabetes mellitus, **colitis**, thyroid disease, inflammatory bowel disease, **Addison's disease**, and certain types of tumors. Patients with these illnesses may present with weight loss, loss of appetite, nausea, vomiting, and growth failure. Malnutrition can result from complications of these conditions. In some patients, these conditions can also precipitate the onset of an eating disorder. Medical conditions that have been associated with an increased risk for developing an eating disorder include diabetes and cystic fibrosis, both of which may be associated with concerns about body image and can require certain dietary restrictions, making it more difficult to manage a co-occurring eating disorder.

Anorexia nervosa can also either mimic or co-occur with psychiatric illnesses. Symptoms such as irritability, worry, social anxiety, social withdrawal, and insomnia are common in eating disorders, just as they are in depression, anxiety, and other mental illnesses. A healthcare professional can help to determine which, if any, coexisting condition(s) may be present and will establish the priorities for treatment.

The following are brief descriptions of psychiatric conditions found to coexist with anorexia nervosa:

- **Depression:** a significant disturbance in mood characterized by such symptoms as tearfulness, social withdrawal, irritability, lack of pleasure, sleeping and eating changes, and low energy levels. *As many as 40–70% of eating disorder patients have co-occurring symptoms of depression.*
- **Anxiety:** a state of worry, fear, apprehension, uneasiness, or distress. Physical symptoms such as dizziness, lightheadedness, or shortness of breath may or may not also occur. **Social phobia** is a form of anxiety where a person avoids certain types of social situations or has increased symptoms of anxiety in those situations.
- **Obsessive-compulsive disorder (OCD):** a form of anxiety consisting of intense, persistent, recurrent, and disturbing thoughts, impulses, and repetitive behaviors. The thoughts (obsessions) are experienced as uncontrollable and cause distress. The repetitive behaviors (compulsions) are often performed with the intent of reducing the distress caused by obsessive thoughts. **Note:** see Question 32 for a description of obsessive-compulsive personality disorder (OCPD), a diagnosis that is distinct from OCD, yet shares a similar name.
- **Body dysmorphic disorder (BDD):** a severe form of body image disturbance characterized by an excessive concern or preoccupation with a perceived defect in one's appearance. This perceived defect may be an exaggerated concern, or it may even be imaginary. Individuals experience intense distress over their appearance and may find their preoccupations difficult to control (see Question 46).

Social phobia

An anxiety disorder that is characterized by a persistent, intense fear of being evaluated, judged, criticized or humiliated in social situations. These fears can be triggered by the real or imagined scrutiny by others. Social phobia can cause extreme distress and may be accompanied by severe blushing, sweating, tearfulness, trembling, nausea, or feelings of panic.

- **Attention deficit hyperactivity disorder (ADHD):** a persistent pattern of inattention and hyperactivity or impulsivity. The inattention may be present in school, work, or social situations. Feelings of restlessness are common. Recent findings suggest girls with ADHD are 2.7 times more likely to develop anorexia than girls without ADHD.

- **Post-traumatic stress disorder (PTSD):** a severe form of anxiety that may develop after experiencing a traumatic, life-threatening, or other very distressing situation. Symptoms can also develop after witnessing an event that involves a threat to another person. Feelings of hopelessness, guilt, despair, shame, or horror may be experienced. Avoidance, mood swings, impulsive behavior, **somatic** complaints, and interpersonal difficulties may be present. In severe cases, a person may experience psychotic symptoms such as hallucinations or paranoia.

- **Personality disorders:** enduring, pervasive, and inflexible patterns of behavior, thought, and interaction with others that cause significant functional impairment or distress. An evaluation of a person's long-term social, interpersonal, cognitive, and personality functioning is essential for an accurate diagnosis. Avoidant personality disorder (see Question 36) and obsessive-compulsive personality disorder (see Question 32) are examples of personality disorders that may co-occur with anorexia.

- **Substance use disorders:** alcohol use, drug use, and/or abuse may also coexist with anorexia.

Somatic

Pertaining to the body.

18. I recently read about the misuse of laxatives and other medications to promote weight loss. What should I know about this weight-loss practice?

Eating disorder patients commonly report the use of, and/or abuse of, various medications, herbs, and over-the-counter

(OTC) products. Used as weight control or purging agents, many of these products can be harmful when taken in a manner inconsistent with their intended use. In addition, young people may mix prescription drugs with other drugs of abuse, such as marijuana and alcohol, putting them at risk for drug interactions and overdose. I have detailed some of the most commonly misused products, including prescription and OTC medications, as well as herbs and vitamin supplements.

Laxatives

Laxatives are the most commonly abused substance by people with anorexia; an estimated 50% of anorexia patients report self-induced vomiting or the abuse of laxatives. Indeed, some states in the United States have restricted the sale of laxatives due to the dangers associated with their abuse. Typically, laxatives are used by eating disorder patients as a means of weight control; however, as with other forms of purging, laxatives are actually *not* an effective means of losing weight. Medical studies have documented that laxatives do not prevent the absorption of calories, nor do they help eliminate fat from the body. Diarrhea that results from laxative use may lead a person to *believe* that weight loss has occurred, but in reality, any weight loss that may follow the use of laxatives is due to the loss of *fluids* and valuable electrolytes, not food, from the body.

Furthermore, the abuse of laxatives can result in **rebound water retention**, leading to the faulty belief that weight gain has occurred, thereby perpetuating the cycle of laxative abuse. **Tolerance** for the drug can develop with prolonged usage, which can result in an increase in use of the drug over time. Prolonged use and abuse of laxatives can have serious physical complications, including painful constipation (as a result of colon impairment), cramping, nausea, fainting, weakness, gastrointestinal bleeding, **rectal prolapse**, **edema**, electrolyte imbalances, cardiac arrhythmias, permanent colon damage, kidney dysfunction, and, in severe cases, kidney failure or sudden death. Certain laxatives are detectable in urine, blood,

Weight Loss and Other Warning Signs

Rebound water retention

Fluid retained by the body after discontinuing diuretic treatment.

Tolerance

Physical or psychological adaptation to the effects of a substance or action, requiring larger amounts to produce the same desired effects.

Rectal prolapse

Protrusion of the rectum (the lowest part of the intestine) through the anal canal.

Edema

An accumulation of excess fluid in the tissues of the body.

or stool samples with a simple test, so parents of children or teens with anorexia can ask their family physician to help determine if laxative abuse is a concern.

Treatment for mild electrolyte fluid imbalance involves at-home mineral supplementation, while more severe, persistent cases can be difficult to correct and may require intravenous mineral fluid and mineral replacement in a hospital setting. The return of normal bowel function may take up to several weeks to resume. Although fluid retention may last for a few days, laxative withdrawal does not cause any permanent weight gain, and any swelling in the abdomen or ankles will likely remit after the body readjusts to normal bowel movements. It is helpful when ceasing the use of laxatives to drink plenty of non-caffeinated fluids, especially water, to increase the daily intake of natural fiber (found in whole grains, fruits, vegetables, and oat bran) and to get regular, non-excessive physical activity, as these measures can promote natural bowel function.

Diuretics

Diuretics are another medication prone to abuse by those with anorexia. Diuretic medications rid the body of excess water by elevating the rate of urine excretion. OTC forms are frequently used by women to reduce water retention associated with the menstrual cycle, and prescription forms are used by patients with high blood pressure, liver cirrhosis, or certain kidney diseases. Unfortunately, in their pursuit of thinness, eating disorder patients may also abuse diuretics. Although fluid loss may give the *appearance* of weight loss, any actual loss is in the form of valuable fluids that are necessary for proper organ functioning. As with laxative abuse, the misuse of diuretics can have serious health-related consequences.

As with laxative abuse, the misuse of diuretics can have serious health-related consequences.

Prescription Medications

According to the National Institute on Drug Abuse, reports of the misuse of prescription medications have increased significantly in the past decade. Some of these occasions of misuse involve inappropriate attempts at weight control. Thyroid medications, asthma medications, and stimulants used to treat attention deficit hyperactivity disorder (ADHD) are examples of medications that may be appropriately prescribed for treatment of a primary medical condition, yet may be misused for weight-loss purposes.

An alarming practice that has gained recent attention involves patients (typically females) with Type I **diabetes mellitus**. An increasing number of these patients are engaging in an extremely risky and harmful weight-loss practice known as "diabulimia." Some patients attempt to purge calories by skipping doses of **insulin**, which causes the body to urinate out **glucose** from the body. However, there is a grave risk of serious complications from this behavior, such as blindness, need for limb amputation, kidney failure, coma, and even death. Despite these risks, more young women who desperately need their life-sustaining insulin are skipping their shots. According to the Associated Press, estimates of diabulimia among women with Type I diabetes in the United States are as high as 450,000, up to one-third of the total number of female diabetics. Some studies put the rate closer to 40%. Warning signs for diabulimia include a change in eating habits (typically eating more while still losing weight), low energy levels, high blood-sugar levels, and frequent urination.

Diet Pills

The recent boom in the diet industry has yielded many new OTC methods of weight loss, many of which can be misused by those with an eating disorder. OTC diet pills are the second most abused substance by those with anorexia. Some of the popular weight-loss ingredients in diet pills include caffeine and Phenyl-propranolamine, an ingredient which can cause insomnia, mood changes, anxiety, irritability, and, in large doses, psychosis, seizures, cerebrovascular hemorrhage (stroke), and kidney failure. In 2000, the Food and Drug Administration (FDA) issued a health advisory

Weight Loss and Other Warning Signs

Diabetes mellitus

A condition or disease in which the body is unable to appropriately control blood-sugar (glucose) levels. The two types of diabetes are referred to as insulin-dependent (Type I) and non-insulin dependent (Type II).

Insulin

A hormone produced by the pancreas that helps the body regulate blood-sugar level.

Glucose

A type of sugar found in the blood and a source of energy for the body.

concerning Phenyl-propranolamine after a Yale study suggested it might have been responsible for hundreds of cases of reported strokes. Likewise, Ephedra (or Ephedrine), was banned by the FDA in 2004 due to the increased risk of heart attack. However, these ingredients still find their way into the medicine cabinets of some who pursue extreme weight loss. (Also watch for a product ingredient called Ma Huang, the Chinese herbal equivalent to Ephedra).

Herbal Diet Products

So called "herbal," or "natural" weight-loss products can be just as dangerous as diet pills made from synthetic ingredients, and many can have serious and potentially lethal side effects. Even caffeine, when taken in extremely large doses, may cause chronic insomnia, breathlessness, persistent anxiety, and mild **delirium**. Here is a list of some herbal agents used for weight loss or as purging agents, along with their potential adverse effects.

Delirium

An acute state of mental confusion with a sudden onset, usually reversible; includes impaired concentration, disorientation, anxiety, and sometimes hallucinations.

Tachycardia

Abnormally rapid heart rate.

- Ephedra: a stimulant that may cause nervousness, dizziness, cardiac arrhythmia, stroke, and sudden death.
- Yohimbine: an appetite suppressant that may cause anxiety, elevated blood pressure, nausea, insomnia, **tachycardia**, tremor, and kidney failure. Yohimbine is also marketed in a number of products for body building and "enhanced male performance."
- Chromium Picolinate: an ingredient in weight-loss products that has been reportedly associated with hypoglycemia, dissolving of muscle tissue, and cognitive and personality disturbances.
- Cascara: used as a laxative and purging agent. May cause severe vomiting, electrolyte imbalance, and cardiac arrhythmia.
- Senna: also a laxative that can cause excessive fluid loss, cramping, and nausea.

Purging Agents and Emetics

Perhaps the most widely reported risk for misuse of an OTC is associated with the **emetic** Ipecac. Found in many home medicine cabinets, Ipecac is an OTC remedy used by some parents to prevent poisoning in children from accidental ingestion of a toxic substance. Ipecac has frequently, and tragically, been misused as a purging agent by eating disorder patients in order to repeatedly induce vomiting. Ipecac is *never* intended to be used without the express supervision of a physician. Even in small, repeated doses, use of this emetic syrup can be fatal. Patients who use Ipecac to induce vomiting can develop an irreversible cardiac condition called myocardial toxicity, or poisoning of the heart muscle. Symptoms of cardio-myopathy include muscle weakness (often severe enough to prevent a person from walking or lifting their head), seizure, irregular heartbeat, blackouts, and respiratory complications. It can take weeks or even months to recover from Ipecac poisoning. Death can occur from the use of Ipecac, as was reportedly the case with the well-known musician Karen Carpenter; the substance caused severe damage to her heart, eventually leading to cardiac arrest and death. It is *essential* to inform your physician if you use, or have ever used, this substance as a purging agent. If no damage to the heart muscle has occurred, full recovery is possible.

Emetic

An agent that induces vomiting.

Ipecac is never *intended to be used without the express supervision of a physician.*

19. What are some of the normal physical and weight changes associated with puberty?

An understanding of normal adolescent development can be helpful, particularly when a young person displays warning signs associated with anorexia. The word *puberty* comes from a Latin word that means "adulthood"; the term is used to describe the time when a child goes through the process of becoming a mature adult. Visible changes occur physically, but puberty is associated with various social, behavioral, and psychological changes as well. Puberty itself is actually a lengthy process, beginning years before a young woman's first menstrual period or the development of secondary sexual characteristics in both boys and girls.

Before any physical signs of puberty can be observed, the production of hormones responsible for sexual maturation begins to increase (in girls, **estrogen** is produced in the ovaries; in boys, **androgens**, such as testosterone, are produced in the testes). This increase in hormone production leads to the development of outward, physical signs of sexual maturity. The process of pubertal change normally begins between ages 8 and 12 in females and between ages 9 and 14 in males. The entire process can take up to four years. During this time, boys and girls typically experience a growth spurt in height. Girls can grow between 8 and 12 inches taller. Likewise, boys gain approximately 20% of their adult height during this stage, sometimes growing 4 to 5 inches in a year's time. Weight gain is also substantial during this time of development. Both boys and girls are expected to gain roughly 50% of their adult weight—that is a doubling of weight within a few years of pubertal onset. This means that a female teenager can commonly gain up to 40–50 pounds in just a few years.

Body shape also changes during puberty. In girls, the hips and thighs widen. Total body fat percentage increases in females (from about 8% to 20–25%) and fat "pads" develop on the stomach, thighs, and buttocks. This increase in body fat is essential for menstruation to begin. In contrast, boys' body fat percentage drops (from about 20–25% to between 10–15%) and muscle mass increases significantly; however, total weight gain in males averages 50% of their adult weight. Your child's physician will routinely plot the growth in height and weight that takes place during puberty. For parents of a child or adolescent with anorexia, growth charts can be helpful for monitoring progress in treatment as measured by a return to normal development (growth charts for home use and reference can be found online at *www.cdc.gov/growthcharts*).

Estrogen

Female hormone produced by the ovaries. It stimulates the development of secondary sexual characteristics and induces menstruation in women.

Androgens

Male sex hormones, responsible for the development of male secondary sex characteristics.

Timing of pubertal development appears to play a role in body dissatisfaction and the development of eating disorders. Studies show that early maturing girls and late maturing boys are at greater risk for body dissatisfaction. Early maturation in girls is associated with poorer self-esteem, increased likelihood of depression, more behavioral problems, and poorer achievement in school; while late maturing boys experience less peer popularity, greater parental conflict, less confidence, and lower school achievement.

To be sure, changes in physical appearance can be a source of stress and anxiety for many teens. Predominant cultural ideas about beauty and attractiveness inundate the average young person at a time when they are typically struggling just to feel comfortable with their changing appearance. Coupled with the expected physical changes, teens face the additional pressure of adjusting to the changing social roles of adolescence. As children begin to look more like adults, responsibilities at school and in the home increase, an interest in dating begins to develop, and decisions about future vocational plans and adult identity loom on the horizon. For these teens, a changing body can become a symbol of the changing expectations and responsibilities associated with adulthood.

Studies show that maturity fears are common among teens and represent an increased risk for anorexia. For some, calorie restriction and weight loss become a false means of remaining physically childlike, thus superficially delaying the arrival of adulthood. Anorexia symptoms may be a means for coping with the demands of maturity while simultaneously allowing teens to "shrink away" or "disappear" from these demands. Some patients report that anorexia provides an illusion of control at a time when uncontrollable bodily changes are taking place. Parents, coaches, and teachers can provide helpful support to young people at this stage of development. Patience, acceptance, and an understanding of the pressures experienced by teens can help vulnerable individuals feel safe in a time of

Weight Loss and Other Warning Signs

great change. Be open to talking with your teen about the changes they are experiencing, but also be sure to give them enough autonomy as they navigate their way through puberty and into adulthood.

20. My daughter recently said she just wants to lose "a little weight" in order to feel better about herself. Should I be concerned?

Many parents echo such concerns. It can be both difficult and confusing to sort through the many mixed messages about the benefits and risks of dieting. On the one hand, parents know that there are proven health benefits to a balanced diet that is low in saturated fats and simple sugars. On the other hand, moms and dads know that attention paid to dieting, weight loss, and body shape can become a preoccupation that leads some kids down a path toward body dissatisfaction and disordered eating.

If your teenager expresses discomfort or dissatisfaction with some aspect of their body shape, they are not alone. In fact, 40–60% of normal weight teens describe themselves as weighing too much. More than 50% of teens exercise to lose weight or improve their body shape, 60% diet regularly, and the majority are preoccupied with their food intake. Alarmingly, in a survey that gave three magic wishes for anything they wanted to girls aged 11 to 17, the number one wish for almost all of them was to lose weight and keep it off!

Alarmingly, in a survey that gave three magic wishes for anything they wanted to girls aged 11 to 17, the number one wish for almost all of them was to lose weight and keep it off!

We know that the prevalence of unhealthy diet behaviors is *unprecedented* in today's society. A 2008 issue of *Self* magazine reported that 65% of American women surveyed between the ages of 25 and 45 report engaging in disordered eating behaviors, and a full 75% endorse some unhealthy thoughts, feelings, or behaviors associated with their bodies, weight, or food intake. In another survey, two out of five women and one out of five men said they would trade three to five years of their life to achieve their weight goals!

Indeed, unhealthy dieting and body image dissatisfaction are commonplace in our society; however, you may not be aware of how early the weight obsession is starting.

- Research shows that dieting to lose weight and fear of fatness are common in girls as young as 7, and 81% of 10-year-old girls say they are afraid of being fat.
- In 1970, the average girl started dieting at age 14; by 1990, the average age dropped to 8. Fifty-one percent of 9- and 10-year-old girls say they feel better about themselves when they are on a diet, and one-half of 4th grade girls are on a diet.
- A 1998 study of 6th to 8th grade boys reported that 4% attempted to lose weight through self-induced vomiting and/or laxative use (Walsh and Cameron 2005).
- Nearly one-half of teenage girls and one-third of teenage boys use unhealthy weight control behaviors such as skipping meals, fasting, smoking cigarettes, vomiting, or taking laxatives.
- A recent study showed that adolescent girls were more afraid of gaining weight than of nuclear war, developing cancer, or losing their parents.

Each year since 1996, more than 40 billion dollars has been spent annually in the United States on diets and diet products. This figure includes money spent on diet centers and diet camps, prepackaged foods, over-the-counter and prescription diet pills, weight-loss books and magazines, commercial fitness centers, sugar-free, fat-free, and reduced calorie food products, imitation fats, sugar substitutes, and other diet-related interventions. Countless billions more are spent on advertising for diet products. However, one thing that advertisers of weight-loss products will *not* tell you: Dieting *can* be dangerous. In fact, recent studies show that unless there is a medical necessity, weight-loss diets may just do more harm than good. Not only can dieting trigger behaviors and attitudes about weight that may progress into a more serious eating disturbance, but

Weight-loss diets may just do more harm than good.

studies show that repeated cycles of losing and gaining weight can have negative, harmful effects on health, such as loss of endurance, decreased oxygen utilization, electrolyte imbalances, weakness, increased risk of heart disease, metabolic changes, and osteoporosis. In addition, medical studies show that dieters have slowed mental reaction time, decreased working memory capacity, and reduced concentration. Chronic dieting has been linked to depression, low self-esteem, anxiety, stress, and increased binge/purge behaviors.

So, if you are concerned by your child's sudden interest in dieting, perhaps you are justified. While dieting can be done safely, it can also pose serious health risks. Moreover, an early interest in dieting can suggest a problem with your child's self-image. Keep in mind, studies show that the risk of developing an eating disorder increases with an earlier age at onset of dieting behaviors.

Sarah shares:

When I was in 8th grade, I went to the doctor's office for a checkup and was told that I was above the 50th percentile for height and weight. I decided that I would be happy with myself if I lost five pounds, and when I lost the weight I honestly did look in the mirror and liked what I saw. But I had developed an incredibly hostile relationship with food to lose just those few pounds, and my diet quickly moved from wanting to lose weight to being terrified of gaining it. I kept restricting, thinking that it would keep me at a constant weight, and even though I didn't like it when I continued to grow thinner, I was unable to face the thought of increasing my calorie intake or gaining any weight back.

21. I read somewhere that restricting calories is good for you and may even be associated with better health and a longer life. So what is wrong with trying a calorie-restricted diet for health-related purposes?

You are probably referring to "Calorie Restriction," also known as CR, a diet plan that emphasizes the reduction of caloric intake, purportedly in the pursuit of "better health." Promoters of this approach emphasize that the focus of CR is not weight loss but the pursuit of a longer life span and the reduction of health problems typically associated with aging. Calorie Restriction proponents base their claims regarding the benefits of CR on research first conducted in the 1930s when a nutritionist from Cornell University accidentally discovered that underfed rats lived longer than rats who were fed a higher calorie diet. While similar results have been found in worms, monkeys, dogs, and other animals, there is no evidence that CR leads to a prolonged lifespan in humans. There has been some evidence that CR may lead to lower blood pressure and lower cholesterol; however, the same results are achieved through a balanced approach to diet and exercise.

Evidence also indicates there are some serious concerns associated with CR, namely an increased risk of serious eating disorders such as anorexia nervosa. Calorie Restriction has also been associated with decreased bone density, high risk of bone fracture, increased sensitivity to cold, anemia, weakness, dizziness, fatigue, lethargy, nausea, constipation, gallstones, irritability, depression, menstrual irregularities, and infertility; the same subset of health risks we find in patients with anorexia. Additionally, studies show that people adhering to a CR diet present many of the same behavioral symptoms associated with anorexia, such as food obsession, decreased sexual drive, and increased sensations of hunger. Although very little is known about the long-term effects of CR on normal-weight individuals, research has shown that individuals with a very low BMI have a higher risk of death. Given the risks associated with CR, a more balanced approach toward enhancing health and longevity—one that does not mimic the dangerous dietary restrictions associated with anorexia nervosa—would be a far better choice.

PART THREE

Risk Factors

What causes anorexia nervosa?

Is it true that most people with anorexia have experienced sexual abuse?

How does the mass media influence ideas about anorexia and eating disorders?

More . . .

22. What causes anorexia nervosa?

This is perhaps one of the most frequently asked questions about anorexia and eating disorders. It is natural, of course, for patients, families, and loved ones to find themselves asking, "how did this happen?" Researchers have spent more than a century trying to answer this important question. What they have determined is that there is no *single* cause of the illness. Instead, we now know that a combination of factors (see Figure 2) can contribute to the development of an eating disorder. The presence of these **risk factors** can increase a person's *vulnerability* to anorexia, and, when combined with triggering life events, they may increase the likelihood of developing the disorder.

Each of the following factors has been shown to contribute to a person's overall risk of developing anorexia nervosa. However, a person can develop anorexia *without* the presence of any of these risk factors. Alternatively, not everyone who evidences these risk factors goes on to develop anorexia. Instead, it is more likely that an interaction between various risk factors and life stressors make up a person's overall risk profile. One important note: Knowing the cause of an eating disorder is *not* a prerequisite for getting help! Even if you are unaware of particular risk factors that apply, do not delay getting help for yourself or for a loved one.

Genetic and Biological Risk Factors

Scientific studies have shown that some individuals may have a **genetic predisposition** toward developing an eating disorder, with some research indicating a **hereditability factor** greater than 50%. Multiple genetic influences (rather than a single, specific gene) appear to combine with environmental factors and lead to an increased risk for the illness. Studies show that people with a family history of anorexia are up to 12 times more likely to develop anorexia. Additionally, studies of identical twins with anorexia also point to a genetic predisposition for the illness. Note, however, that not every

Risk factor

A characteristic that increases an individual's likelihood of developing an illness.

An interaction between various risk factors and life stressors make up a person's overall risk profile.

Genetic predisposition

An inherited genetic pattern that may make a person more susceptible to a disease or condition.

Hereditability factor

A calculation of the contribution made by genes to the causation of a disorder or disease.

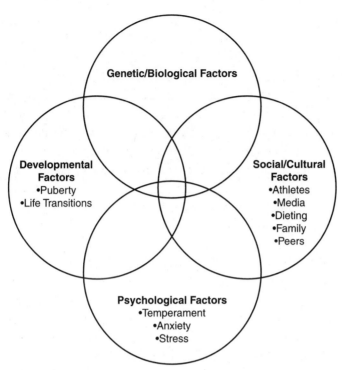

Figure 2   Anorexia Risk Factors

anorexia patient has a family history of eating disorders. According to the University of Maryland Medical Center, only about one-fifth of those with anorexia have a relative with an eating disorder.

Another area of biology that is important in understanding anorexia risk is brain chemistry. Scientific investigations have shown that the regulation of certain brain chemicals, called **neurotransmitters,** play an important role in certain psychiatric illnesses, such as depression and anxiety disorders. While we are just beginning the search into the role these chemicals may play in anorexia, there is increasing evidence that suggests neurotransmitters are a contributing factor in the course of anorexia. Some of the same neurotransmitters that influence aspects of mood and behavior (including **serotonin, norepinephrine,** and **dopamine**) are being investigated as keys to understanding anorexia. A technique called **neuroimaging**

Risk Factors

Neurotransmitter

A chemical substance in the brain that facilitates communication between nerve cells.

Serotonin

A brain chemical thought to be important for regulating sleep, appetite, mood, and pain inhibition.

Norepinephrine

A neurotransmitter in the brain that is involved in the regulation of sleep, arousal, mood, and response to stressful stimuli.

Dopamine

A neurotransmitter which has been associated with the areas of the brain that regulate movement, mood, emotion, motivation, and pleasure.

Neuroimaging

Techniques that allow mapping of the structure or function of the brain.

Functional magnetic resonance imaging (fMRI)

A type of brain scan used to study activity in the brain. An fMRI shows which structures are active during particular mental operations.

Leptin

A protein hormone that helps the body regulate appetite and the metabolism of fats.

Ghrelin

A hormone that relays messages between the digestive system and the brain to stimulate appetite.

Prenatal

Occurring or existing before birth.

Research tells us that anorexia nervosa is a brain disease *with severe metabolic effects on the entire body.*

has allowed scientists to examine the influence of these brain chemicals on human behavior, as well as upon sensations such as hunger and thirst. Neuroimaging was also involved in another recent discovery that revealed female anorexia patients have differences in a part of the brain called the insula, an area important in recognizing taste and responding to pleasure associated with food. Using **functional magnetic resonance imaging (fMRI)** to measure the brain's reaction to taste, researchers from the University of Pittsburgh and the University of California, San Diego, found that individuals with anorexia process taste in a different way than those without an eating disorder.

Multiple areas of biological research have yielded additional advances in the understanding of anorexia. For example, certain digestive hormones (e.g., **leptin** and **ghrelin**) have been found at abnormal levels in anorexia patients. Also, it appears various hormones released in the body during times of stress may play a role. Recent research published in the *Archives of General Psychiatry* further suggests **prenatal** conditions may influence the likelihood of developing anorexia. Thus, as you can well imagine, the biological aspects of anorexia are complex, and research in this area is still in its infancy. We are continually learning more about the interaction between biological and genetic components with other factors that may contribute to the development and course of anorexia. Experts are encouraged by recent research that has lead to the definitive understanding that anorexia is a biological, as well as a behavioral, illness. Thomas Insel, MD, Director of the National Institute of Mental Health, conveyed that understanding when he made this landmark statement in October, 2006:

> *Anorexia Nervosa, among the most serious of mental disorders, can be deadly for young women who get caught up in the malignant cycle of weight loss and compulsive behaviors. . . . Research tells us that anorexia nervosa is a* brain disease *with severe metabolic effects*

on the entire body. While the symptoms are behavioral, this illness has a biological core, with genetic compo- nents, changes in brain activity, and neural pathways currently under study. (emphasis added)

As our understanding of anorexia continues to advance, we find that research not only helps to clarify the nature of this illness but also provides critical support for continued health- care research and the development of more effective means of treatment.

Developmental Factors

Although anorexia can occur throughout the lifespan, the most common period of onset is adolescence. Developmental changes that occur with puberty can increase a youth's atten- tion to, and dissatisfaction with, his or her body image. For both boys and girls, the interaction of pubertal hormonal changes, body preoccupation, and experimental dieting can interact to increase vulnerability to anorexic behaviors. How- ever, while boys tend to gain muscle and lose fat at puberty, girls experience a normal increase in body fat, which is neces- sary for menstruation to occur (see Question 19). This natural increase in body fat may be perceived by some as "getting fat," resulting in attempts at weight control or weight loss. Several studies indicate girls who experience early puberty are at greater risk for an eating disorder.

Peer factors during adolescence may also contribute to an- orexia risk. Boys and girls who experience teasing about ap- pearance and weight have been shown to be at greater risk for eating disorders. Sexual anxieties, unwanted sexual advances, and/or sexual assault have been reported in a significant num- ber of teens with anorexia. Studies suggest peer weight-loss behaviors and dietary restriction among close friends can also have an influence on attitudes about food and weight in adolescents and young adults. Life transitions within this stage of development, such as starting high school, the onset of dating, or leaving home to go to college, may interact with other risk factors to trigger eating disorder behaviors in vulnerable individuals.

Psychological Factors

Multiple psychological factors may contribute to the onset of anorexia. For example, anorexia patients have reported certain general characteristics such as low self-esteem, feelings of inadequacy, anger, guilt, and loneliness. More specific findings include those from a series of studies that revealed two factors distinguishing anorexia patients from other study participants: negative self-evaluation (thinking negatively about oneself) and perfectionism (Fairburn et al. 1999). Certain personality traits have commonly been observed in anorexia patients, though it is important to note that there is no "personality formula" for understanding anorexia, nor is a patient's personality to blame for their illness. Additionally, we are not be able to discern within some research results which observed behaviors may have been a precursor to the development of anorexia and which arose after the onset of the illness. With these caveats in mind, common characteristics have been observed in anorexia patients. These include:

- Perfectionism and extreme conscientiousness
- Fearful or anxious temperament
- Drive for thinness
- Excessive control of emotions
- Sense of personal ineffectiveness or inadequacy
- Difficulty identifying or describing their own feelings
- Obsessive tendencies
- Extreme compliance to the demands of others (an extreme "people pleaser")
- "Harm avoidance" (not wanting to upset anyone by their own behavior)
- Negative body image
- Maturity fears (fears about growing up to adulthood)
- Extreme shyness or social anxiety

- Cognitive inflexibility (rigidity in thinking; "all-or-nothing" thinking)
- Identity concerns
- Social isolation or fear of intimacy

To be clear, no single trait listed here is considered a direct cause for anorexia, nor do all individuals who evidence these traits go on to develop the illness. Rather, it is likely that certain personal characteristics, when combined with other risk factors, may increase one's vulnerability to eating disorders. Other psychological factors that may increase vulnerability are:

- A history of, or a co-occurring, psychological disorder
- Past experience of a traumatic event
- Emotional or interpersonal conflict
- Physical or sexual abuse
- A history of weight concern or childhood obesity
- Childhood feeding problems
- The effects of chronic illness

Occupational Factors, Athletics, and Other Activities

Studies show certain activities that include an emphasis on slenderness or weight control are associated with a higher risk for anorexia. For example, the prevalence rate of anorexia nervosa in ballet dancers is 4 to 25 times higher than that of the general population (Walsh and Cameron 2005). Other sports such as gymnastics, figure skating, wrestling, rowing, swimming, jockeying, track and field, and bodybuilding can involve certain weight restrictions that may lead to unhealthy attempts at weight control. Models and entertainment personalities may also experience social and occupational pressures to be thin. The more a person is involved in these types of activities, especially at advanced levels, the more likely they are to experience pressure about body shape and weight (see Questions 39–41).

Risk Factors

Familial Factors

Over the past several decades, certain commonalities with regard to family considerations have been noted in eating disorders literature. Many of these speculations have gone unsupported by scientific study, while others have proven to have some validity. One point that deserves emphasis is that the family does not *cause* anorexia. Rather, the familial component of a person's experience is another area that can be important in understanding the overall picture of a person's issues with weight and food. To be sure, the way parents interact with their children can have an impact on their emotional development. Yet there is no "type" of family that causes anorexia and, as is true with individual psychological characteristics, we do not know for sure if certain family dynamics are present before an eating disorder develops, or in response to them.

There is a greater risk of someone developing anorexia when another member of the family has had an eating disorder.

Here is what we do know: There is a greater risk of someone developing anorexia when another member of the family has had an eating disorder. This may be due to genetic influences and/or learned behavior within the family environment. For example, parents who have body image issues or unhealthy eating habits of their own may unwittingly make negative comments about weight and appearance that can influence other members of the family. We also know that people who feel less secure or unsafe in their family environment may be at greater risk for an eating disorder. For example, a family history of alcohol or substance abuse, physical, emotional, or sexual abuse, mental illness, or high parental conflict have been shown to increase risk. There is greater speculation, however, about the role of other family characteristics in overall anorexia risk. For example, it has been suggested that parental indifference, extreme over-protectiveness, excessive performance demands, and emotional rigidity may be potential risk factors for a variety of mental illnesses and emotional distress; while compassion, acceptance, encouragement, and nurturing have been associated with greater resilience.

Dieting and Weight Loss Factors

Studies show that most cases of anorexia are preceded by an episode of dieting that progresses to anorexic food restriction and self-starvation. Clearly, not all attempts at dieting lead to disordered eating; however, studies have shown that the risk of developing an eating disorder is higher in dieting than in non-dieting adolescent girls. For example, a 1999 study in the *British Medical Journal* reported that girls who were defined as severe dieters were 18 times more likely than non-dieters to develop an eating disorder within 6 months. Additionally, according to the National Eating Disorders Association, 35% of "normal dieters" gradually progress to pathological dieting, and of those, 20–25% later progress to either sub-clinical or clinical eating disorders. Nonetheless, questions remain regarding the exact nature of the link between dieting and anorexia. Does dieting serve as a trigger for anorexia? Is it dissatisfaction with one's body, and not the act of dieting per se, which represents the greater risk? Does calorie restriction cause physiological changes that lead to eating pathology in at-risk individuals? Does dieting represent a true risk for anorexia, or is it merely an early symptom of the illness? While the exact nature of the relationship between dieting and anorexia is still under investigation, researchers are certain it cannot be ignored.

Thirty-five percent of "normal dieters" gradually progress to pathological dieting, and of those, 20–25% later progress to either sub-clinical or clinical eating disorders.

Social/Cultural Factors

In addition to individual factors such as genetics, family experience, and personality factors, certain social and cultural factors may increase the risk of developing anorexia nervosa. For example, recent research suggests Western cultural influences may play a role in the overall picture of eating disorders risk. Central to this influence is the value placed in Western societies on appearance, beauty, and the pursuit of thinness. Some experts even go so far as to say the preoccupation with weight and body image displayed in anorexia patients is merely an "exaggerated reflection" of the ubiquitous pursuit of thinness that pervades our Western culture. Even the casual observer

Risk Factors

would agree that ours is a culture that values thinness. One can scarcely pass a magazine rack, turn on the television, or watch popular films without being bombarded with images and ideas that equate success, happiness, and social acceptance with the **"thin ideal."** Eating disorders experts believe cultural expectations such as these have a profound effect on the prevalence of anorexia in Western society. Indeed, anorexia is often referred to as a "culture-bound syndrome," implying that prevalence of the illness is directly influenced by attitudes, values, and behaviors that are prized in Western culture.

Studies show anorexia nervosa is most prevalent in industrialized countries where dieting and the pursuit of thinness are the accepted norm. In contrast, non-Western countries report lower rates of anorexia. Researchers are finding that with globalization and Western influence come the desire to emulate Western ideals, including ideals related to appearance and attractiveness. Results of a landmark study published in 1999 revealed a dramatic increase in the rate of eating disorders among teenage girls in the Pacific Island nation of Fiji that was linked to the introduction of Western television programming. Harvard eating disorders researcher Anne Becker studied the eating habits of Fijian schoolgirls between 1995 and 1998, a period that marked the introduction of Western television programming to an otherwise traditional, agricultural society. There was only one TV station available, which broadcasted mostly American, Australian, and British favorites such as *Seinfeld, ER,* and *Melrose Place.* Becker reports that the proportion of students who scored high on an eating disorders risk evaluation rose from 13% to 29% in the 38 months that followed the introduction of TV programming. Those who watched TV at least 3 nights per week were 50% more likely to see themselves as "too fat" and 30% more likely to diet. Fifteen percent had reported they induced vomiting as a means of weight control, up from 3% shortly after the study began. Overall, symptoms of eating disorders among teenage girls increased fivefold in 4 years. A 2005 study of more than

Thin ideal

Cultural attitudes which imply that extreme thinness is a requisite for attractiveness. Such ideas may inadvertently promote unhealthy weight control methods in society-at-large by promoting conformity to an unrealistic "ideal" body shape and size.

Anorexia nervosa is most prevalent in industrialized countries where dieting and the pursuit of thinness are the accepted norm.

100 female international students from Japan, China, Taiwan, and Hong Kong found that a greater acceptance of a Western ideal of thinness was associated with greater eating disorder symptoms. Likewise, a 2007 study published in the *Journal of Nervous and Mental Disease* found that media exposure and travel abroad was correlated with eating disorder symptoms in females from the East African country of Tanzania. Additional studies reported in the *International Journal of Eating Disorders* reveal that as adolescents from more weight-tolerant countries become assimilated to Western culture, they report more fear of weight gain and an increase in symptoms of disordered eating.

Cultural influences of a social nature may also contribute to the increased risk of anorexia among females. According to the *Clinical Manual of Eating Disorders*, the disparity in prevalence rates between male and female adolescents who develop anorexia has been attributed in part to the greater cultural pressures on young women to be thin. Researchers note that appearance is often a central factor to how females are valued in Western culture. Therefore, beauty and body image become more salient to a young woman's self-esteem. In addition, researchers suggest anorexia may be a response to role-conflicts and complex pressures of socialization experienced by contemporary females. A 2003 issue of *Parade* magazine included this comment about the cultural demands placed on women: "In order for a woman to consider herself happy, she has to be in a good relationship, be happy with her kids, her friends have to like her, her job has to be going well, her house has to look good, and she *has to be* thin" (emphasis added). Mounting social and cultural pressures may be just one more piece in the overall puzzle that determines eating disorders risk in vulnerable individuals.

Stress Factors and Emotional "Triggers"

Each of the factors discussed so far can influence an individual's risk of developing an eating disorder. Yet eating disorders are also often precipitated by (or "triggered" by) an emotional life event or period of significant stress. Significant stress, when coupled with inadequate coping resources, can combine with other risk factors to increase a person's vulnerability to illness. Potential triggers for anorexia can include:

- Environmental changes (changes in school, moving to a new home or city)
- Family changes (parental divorce, birth of a child, increased familial stress)
- Loss of a loved one (through death or break-up of a relationship)
- Trauma
- Uncomfortable feelings about adult sexuality or unwanted sexual advances
- Maturity fears
- Increased familial responsibility and caretaking
- Dieting to promote weight loss (often for an upcoming special event)
- Industry pressure to maintain a certain physical appearance
- Teasing or being bullied
- Rejection
- Threats to physical safety or security
- Academic difficulties
- Peer pressure (including pressure from team sports)
- Chronic illness, especially one that may affect weight or appearance
- Other significant loss or disappointment

23. Is it true that most people with anorexia have experienced sexual abuse?

Approximately 30% of females with anorexia (and up to 65% of all eating disorder patients) report a history of childhood sexual abuse—a percentage comparable to the rate of sexual abuse reported by patients with other psychiatric illnesses. Some studies report that sexual abuse history is higher among patients who binge/purge than among patients with restrict-ing-type anorexia. Sexual abuse, sexual harassment, and other sources of trauma are considered a risk factor for disordered eating and body image disturbance; however, a history of sexual abuse is not seen in all patients with eating disorders, and conversely, not everyone with a history of sexual abuse will go on to develop anorexia or another eating disorder.

24. How does the mass media influence ideas about anorexia and eating disorders?

Media images and advertising messages about weight and appearance are certainly hard to ignore (see Exhibit 6). These days, fast-paced music videos, glossy fashion magazines, and cutting-edge television programs are a normal part of routine American life. A reflection of our culture's thin obsession, television "news-magazines," such as *Entertainment Tonight* and *Access Hollywood* regularly feature stories about the latest "celebrity slim-down." Popular film and television celebrities on the red carpet seem to be slimmer each year as they show-case high-fashion designers and couture clothing. Tabloid stories repeatedly reinforce a standard of beauty that em-phasizes thinness and dress size over health and well-being, equating fashion chic with a dangerously thin waistline. Just walk by a magazine stand in your local bookstore and chances are you will be bombarded with images of thin, sometimes gaunt looking models surrounded by eye-catching phrases such as "ultimate weight-loss secrets!" "10 weeks to a slimmer, better you!" or "lose those last 10 pounds for good!" Likewise, advertisements in magazines and on television routinely pair images of thin, attractive people in order to sell products. Unfortunately, we know from scientific studies that repeated exposure to waif-thin models and images that promote a thin ideal have a negative effect on those who view these images and internalize such body ideals.

Studies show that the standards of beauty portrayed through the media have ushered in an ever-increasing thin ideal over

> ### Exhibit 6   Facts About Media Influence
>
> Few would deny that ours is a culture that receives a vast amount of input from the mass media. But did you know:
>
> - The average person living in the United States is exposed to more than 3000 advertising messages per day.
> - The main source of health information for adolescent girls comes from the media.
> - Sixty percent of Caucasian, middle-school-aged girls read at least one fashion magazine regularly.
> - The average adolescent watches 3–4 hours of television per day.
> - The average teenager spends more than 16 hours per week online, and 50% of teens are online every day.
> - One of every 3.8 television commercials sends a message about attractiveness, meaning the average adolescent receives more than 5200 "attractiveness messages" per year.
> - A 20-year review of 1 teen magazine found that in articles that focused on fitness and exercise, 74% encouraged adolescent girls to exercise to become more attractive, and 51% emphasized exercise in order to lose weight. Only rarely were the health benefits of exercise the focus of such articles.
> - Several studies suggest that young women consider fashion magazines and television at least moderately important as a source of information about beauty, nutrition, weight management, and fitness. (Levine and Smolak 1998)

the past several decades. For example, 20 years ago the average female model weighed 8% less than the average American woman; today the average model weighs 23% less than the average woman and is thinner than 98% of American women. The prevailing standards of weight and body shape are virtually unattainable by the average person.

In her book *The Body Myth: Adult Women and the Pressure to Be Perfect*, psychologist and author Margo Maine draws attention to the changing cultural ideals of beauty over the past century. Maine observes that fashion icons of the 1950s included women like Marilyn Monroe, Lana Turner, Sophia Loren, and Jane Russell. Voluptuous women with "curvy" figures were representations of glamour and beauty. In the

1960s, the beauty ideal took a different shape, highlighting the "waif" look of British model Twiggy. The 1980s and 1990s followed with an ever-increasing emphasis on body shape. No longer was the average woman represented on the pages of fashion magazines. Instead, an ultra-thin ideal began to take shape in fashion and entertainment—an image not only unattainable by most U.S. women, but also by many of the women in the photos themselves! Take for example a recent promotional photo from CBS television that featured Katie Couric; from the time she posed for the original photo to the time the promotional photo appeared, Couric's image had been digitally altered to make her appear 20 pounds lighter and 3 dress-sizes smaller! Techniques like this are a normal part of the fashion industry; however, the average consumer may not realize that tens of thousands of dollars are often spent "enhancing" the bodies that grace the pages of their favorite fashion magazines. Even famous celebrities are not immune to the insecurities created by our thin-obsessed culture. Increasingly, notable entertainment personalities have been coming forward to discuss their own struggles with anorexia and other eating disorders in an effort to combat the illnesses and send a positive message to their fans.

The mass media's trend toward increasing thinness has not gone unnoticed by the average American. In 2002, America Online (AOL) conducted a survey in which they asked participants, "What do you think is responsible for many women's poor self-images?" A full 66% selected the response "impossibly beautiful media images." A recent study found that the more frequently young girls read fashion magazines, the more likely they were to diet and to feel that these magazines influenced their ideas about ideal weight and body shape. Nearly half of this study's participants reported wanting to lose weight because of a magazine image, although only 29% were actually overweight (Kilbourne 1999). In addition, studies at both Stanford University and the University of Massachusetts found that 70% of college women say they feel worse about their appearance after reading women's magazines, and 80% of those responding to a survey in *People* magazine stated that images of women on television and in film make them feel insecure about their appearance. Our culture's bias toward extreme thinness has had this effect: 80% of women (four out of every five!) are dissatisfied with their appearance.

The consensus from the literature is this: Mass media exposure has an effect on body image disturbance; negative body image, in turn, has been shown to be a risk factor for disordered eating. Additionally, the negative effects of media exposure may have a long-term effect. A recent study found that adolescent girls who were exposed to television commercials depicting thin, attractive models reported feeling more dissatisfied with their bodies and expressed a greater drive for thinness *up to two years* later. Important to our discussion of anorexia, some studies suggest that the negative effects of media exposure are greater for those at increased risk for the illness. For example, a study published in the *Journal of Social and Clinical Psychology* found that a 15-month subscription to a fashion magazine resulted in increased body dissatisfaction, dieting, and binge/purge symptoms—but only for girls who were considered to have increased risk for an eating disorder prior to the study.

It should be noted that not all studies have found conclusive evidence for a *direct* impact of media images on disordered eating, suggesting that the relationship between the two may not be clear-cut. Therefore, we must stop short of saying that the mass media *directly causes* anorexia. However, we do see a clear connection between a mass media saturated with images of thinness and unhealthy attitudes about weight, body shape, and food. Thus, altogether it appears exposure to media images of the thin-ideal can be considered an additional risk factor that, when combined with the effects of other known risks, may increase an individual's susceptibility to anorexia and other eating disorders.

Male Images in the Media

Studies show that men are not immune to the effect of the media's ideal images of body shape and appearance. Just over a decade ago, there were scarcely any magazines devoted to men's fitness and nutrition. Today, there are more than 20. Researchers are beginning to witness the effect of increasingly muscular male media images on levels of body satisfaction. For example, researchers at the University of Central Florida released a study in 2004 that showed that men who watched television commercials depicting muscular actors reported being unsatisfied with their own physique. Other research has highlighted some of the effects of the fastest growing segment of the entertainment market: video games. One study found that boys who read popular video game magazines containing very muscular characters reported greater body dissatisfaction than boys who read sports, fitness, and even fashion magazines! Men who report body dissatisfaction are more likely, researchers have found, to take protein supplements, display symptoms of an eating disorder, and to think about using steroids to enhance their muscle growth. This preoccupation with muscle growth can lead to a condition called "**muscle dysmorphia**" (sometimes referred to as "reverse anorexia").

A Thin Line on the Catwalk

The fashion industry has also received renewed criticism in recent months for the perceived pressure that designers and modeling agencies place on thinness. The death of two models in 2006 from anorexia, Uruguayan model Luisel Ramos and Brazilian model Ana Carolina Reston, served as wakeup calls regarding the dangers of disordered eating and the prevalence of unhealthy behaviors practiced by some models to be runway ready. These events led many in the eating disorders field to call for stricter standards regarding body weight and for industry guidelines for minimum health requirements. For example, the Academy of Eating Disorders, the National Eating Disorders Association, and the Eating Disorders Coalition all joined together to take a proactive role in trying to reshape the

Risk Factors

Muscle dysmorphia
A condition in which a person becomes fixated on the idea that he or she is not muscular enough and is inordinately preoccupied with thoughts concerning appearance, especially musculature.

health and wellness guidelines of the fashion industry. Among the recommendations were yearly medical exams for models, including eating disorders assessments when appropriate, and the discouragement of all non-healthy weight control behaviors throughout the industry. In the months following these efforts, we have witnessed some initial, positive dialogue between health professionals, eating disorders experts, and fashion designers. In the fall of 2006, the organizers of Madrid Fashion Week decided to ban underweight models from the runways in an attempt to promote a healthier image of the fashion industry; a full 30% of the models were turned away for being underweight! In July 2008, German fashion industry representatives likewise signed a voluntary agreement to ban underweight models from their fashion shows. You can view the Academy of Eating Disorder sponsored Guidelines for the Fashion Industry on their Web site at *www.aedweb.org*.

Sarah shares:

Throughout my battle with anorexia, it was hard to ignore the tempting weight-loss solutions offered on the covers of nearly every magazine. With or without meaning to, I soaked up the information from each of these magazines, and before long I was a walking weight-loss connoisseur.

Regarding the statistic that 80% of women are dissatisfied with their appearance: A therapist of mine once described warped American beauty ideals using the term "normative discontent." In our culture, the average person wants to lose weight, discussing diets is the norm, and nearly everyone's natural appearance is seen to have weaknesses.

In addition, not only are extremely thin stars portrayed as "fit" and "healthy," but truly healthy stars are described as "voluptuous" or "curvy"—words that, in my disordered mind, simply meant "fat" and "out of control."

25. What about information on the Internet? Are Web sites about anorexia helpful or harmful?

The good news about online health information is that the Internet can indeed be a useful tool for better understanding anorexia, learning about treatment options, and locating community support. Proactive eating disorders organizations such as the Academy for Eating Disorders (AED), the National Association for Anorexia Nervosa and Associated Disorders (ANAD), and the National Eating Disorders Association (NEDA) maintain helpful Web sites that provide information and resources for anorexia patients and their loved ones, as well as for the public (see Appendix B for helpful Web sites). The Internet is also fast becoming a treatment tool. Although research in this area is limited, preliminary results show that certain forms of Internet-based intervention may provide a future complement to traditional face-to-face treatments.

Unfortunately, while there are many Internet sites that offer practical and helpful information about anorexia, there are also numerous Web sites that host just the opposite, offering information that is inaccurate, misleading, and even dangerous. The past decade has witnessed a surge of popularity in a genre of Web sites referred to as "Pro-Ana" (pro-anorexia) and "Pro-Mia" (pro-bulimia) in their content (Shepphird 2007). Users and hosts alike are predominantly teenage girls who engage in unhealthy dialogue about anorexia nervosa, body image, and other issues related to disordered eating. Alarmingly, one of the main ideas promoted on these Web sites is that anorexia is a lifestyle choice, not an illness. Eating disorders are heralded as a means of achieving "perfection," and attempts are made to aid others in disordered behaviors by providing information about purging agents, ideas for severely restricting food intake, and "tips" for "staying strong" in the quest for the "perfect" body. Slogans, poems, personal stories, and photographs of dangerously underweight women and men are offered to visitors as "thin-spiration" for

Risk Factors

anorexic behaviors (see Exhibit 7). Hosts and visitors alike share thoughts on ways to keep their behaviors hidden from loved ones, oppose intervention from healthcare professionals, and refuse family involvement in recovery. The proliferation of these Web sites is of great concern. In addition, Pro-Ana content is popping up on popular social networking sites such as MySpace and Facebook, technologies used by upwards of 80–96% of all 12- to 17-year-olds.

A recent study published in the medical journal *Pediatrics* showed that teens looking for eating disorders information on the Internet are more likely to be hospitalized for their condition than teens who do not seek such information online. Results of a 2007 study published in the *International Journal of Eating Disorders* found that after just *a single viewing* of a pro-anorexia Web site, participants reported lower self-esteem, perceived themselves as heavier, and said they were more likely to think about their weight in the near future.

For many visitors, these Web sites can create an artificial sense of community by offering a seductive sense of camaraderie and belonging. They encourage users to wear solidarity bracelets to affirm their "membership" in the pro-eating disorders community: a red bracelet for anorexia, purple for bulimia, and green for EDNOS (see Question 3 for more about EDNOS). One site welcomes visitors with warm comments such as, "Good luck! Hugs and kisses," and one user writes, "This is truly one of the most accepting, close-knit communities of any on the net." "Please Ana [a reference to anorexia], don't give up on me," states a Pro-Ana blogger, "all that's important is that you love me. Today, I renew our friendship and resolve to be faithful to you."

In February 2008, in the United Kingdom, 40 Members of Parliament signed a motion urging government action against Pro-Ana sites. The motion was timed to coincide with the U.K. National Eating Disorder Awareness Week. In April 2008, a French bill was introduced that would outlaw material that

---

Exhibit 7   Pro-Anorexia Web Site Content

Many of the pro-anorexia Web sites share certain features, two of which are "Ana's Creed," eight beliefs subscribed to by pro-anorexia Web hosts, and the "Thin Commandments," a set of ten "rules" to follow for achieving an anorexic "lifestyle."

Ana's Creed

- I believe in Control, the only force mighty enough to bring order to the chaos that is my world.
- I believe that I am the most vile, worthless, and useless person ever to have existed on the planet and that I am totally unworthy of anyone's time and attention.
- I believe that other people who tell me differently are idiots. If they could see how I really am, then they would hate me almost as much as I do.
- I believe in perfection and strive to attain it.
- I believe in salvation through trying just a bit harder than I did yesterday.
- I believe in bathroom scales as an indicator of my daily successes and failures.
- I believe in hell because I sometimes think that I am living in it.
- I believe in a wholly black and white world, the losing of weight, recrimination for sins, abnegation of the body, and a life ever-fasting.

The Thin Commandments

- If you are not thin, you aren't attractive.
- Being thin is more important than being healthy.
- You must buy clothes, cut your hair, take laxatives, starve yourself, and do anything to make yourself look thinner.
- Thou shall not eat without feeling guilty.
- Thou shall not eat fattening food without punishing oneself afterwards.
- Thou shall count calories and restrict intake accordingly.
- What the scale says is the most important thing.
- Losing weight is good; gaining weight is bad.
- You can never be too thin.
- Being thin and not eating are signs of true will power and success.

"provokes a person to seek excessive thinness by encouraging prolonged restriction of nourishment." In America, organizations such as ANAD have had some limited success removing pro-anorexia Web sites from Internet search engines.

For parents and loved ones, there are ways to minimize the negative effect of these sites. First, if you suspect that your child may be involved in the pro-anorexia movement, talk openly about it. Ask questions about the sites your kids visit online. Inform any Pro-Ana Web site users in your family about Web sites that promote recovery from eating disorders as a healthy alternative. These Web sites have been a source of support for those recovering after being a part of the pro-anorexia community. Two of these Web sites are *www. WeBiteBack.com* and *www.UnitedWeStarveNoMore.com*. Second, parents with teens at high risk for an eating disorder may want to consider utilizing Internet parental controls, in the same way that you might block Web sites with adult content from your home computer. You may wish to keep home computers in a common area to monitor online activity. Studies show that three-fourths of teens report that their parents "almost never" monitor the Web sites they use or the time they spend online, and one-third of teens report that their parents know "very little" about what they do on the Internet. Third, be sure to stay involved in your child's recovery, be informed, maintain open dialogue about your child's need for community, and promote healthy ways of building self-esteem. Fourth, while the Internet can be a useful tool for locating eating disorders recovery resources in your community, it is important to distinguish between accurate, helpful information and information that can have a detrimental effect. If you are unsure of the accuracy of any anorexia information you find online, ask your healthcare professional.

26. Does substance abuse commonly co-occur with eating disorders such as anorexia?

"For many young women, eating disorders like anorexia and bulimia are joined at the hip with smoking, binge drinking, and illicit drug use," states Joseph A. Califano, Jr., the former U.S. Secretary of Health, Education, and Welfare. Indeed, scientific studies confirm that substance abuse and eating disorders do appear to be closely linked. A 2004 review conducted by The National Center on Addiction and Substance Abuse (CASA) at Columbia University revealed that up to one-half of individuals with an eating disorder abuse alcohol or illicit drugs. However, studies show that there is a lower rate of drug and alcohol abuse among patients with anorexia nervosa than with some other eating disorders. According to the *Clinical Manual of Eating Disorders*, the rate of substance-related disorders among anorexia patients ranges between 10–33%. The risk is reportedly higher among anorexia patients with the binge/purge subtype than among restricting-type anorexia patients.

The CASA report points to shared risk factors that exist both for substance abuse as well as for eating disorders. These factors include life stressors, family history, mood disorders, low self-esteem, social pressures, and susceptibility to messages from advertising and the media. In addition, the report notes shared characteristics of the two afflictions, namely secretiveness, social isolation, compulsive behaviors, and the life threatening nature of both conditions. Substances that pose the greatest risk for abuse among eating disorder patients are caffeine, tobacco, alcohol, diuretics, laxatives, emetics, **amphetamines**, cocaine, and heroin.

27. Sometimes I have an extremely difficult time communicating my emotions. Could this problem be related to my anorexia?

You may be referring to **alexithymia**, a trait characterized by the inability to identify and describe emotions, confusion about one's own feelings, and/or an apparent lack of consideration about one's own personal experiences. Literally translated, the word alexithymia means "absence of words for emotion," a fitting description for those who experience it. Although people with alexithymia experience the expected *physical* responses associated with emotions, such as changes in heart rate, or even tears, they are typically unable to connect these reactions to their underlying emotions. Moreover,

Amphetamines
A class of drugs that has a stimulant effect on the central nervous system of the body.

Risk Factors

while some people with alexithymia may be able to express that they feel certain *sensations*, such as sadness, fear, happiness, or anger, they are typically unable to connect these sensations to a particular event or circumstance. Alexithymia is *not* the same thing as apathy, *denial* of emotion, or a lack of concern for others. However, a person with alexithymia may appear emotionally detached and may have difficulties connecting to others.

Studies show that rates of alexithymia are higher among those with eating disorders than among the general population. Research published in *Comprehensive Psychiatry* reported that approximately 40–68% of eating disorder patients experience some degree of alexithymia. Alexithymia is also common among people with depression and certain types of anxiety disorders. While more research is needed, the inability to regulate uncomfortable emotions coupled with a lessened ability to experience positive emotions (both are associated with alexithymia) may contribute to the overall risk of developing anorexia.

Approximately 40–68% of eating disorder patients experience some degree of alexithymia.

The causes of alexithymia are still under investigation. Some studies indicate that alexithymia may be due to a disturbance in the right hemisphere of the brain, an area largely responsible for processing emotional cues. Other studies suggest a decreased ability for neural communication between the various regions of the brain involved in translating emotional cues and expressing emotions. Some researchers have looked at the importance of parental response to their children's emotions and the effect this may have on a child's natural range of expressing emotion.

Externally oriented thinking

Thinking that tends to focus on external events rather than inner emotional experiences.

Healthcare professionals typically assess for alexithymia using an inventory called the Toronto Alexithymia Scale-20, which measures three core features: difficulty identifying feelings, difficulty communicating feelings, and **externally oriented thinking**. This brief screening tool can help determine the degree to which alexithymia may affect treatment and recovery from anorexia. Problem solving therapy and Dialectical Behavior Therapy (see Question 83) are two therapeutic approaches that have shown promise with alexithymia. Alexithymia can pose a challenge to recovery, especially if it goes unnoticed, so be sure to talk to your healthcare professional if you experience any of the following signs of alexithymia:

- Difficulty identifying and/or verbalizing different types of feelings
- Difficulty distinguishing between emotional feelings and bodily sensations
- Limited understanding of what causes unique feelings
- Limited fantasy thinking or emotional content of imagination
- Lack of enjoyment and pleasure-seeking
- Often perceived by others as excessively logical, or unsentimental
- Often confused by others' emotional reactions

Sarah shares:

Even to this day, I sometimes find myself using food restriction or compulsive exercising as a distraction from the bigger issues in my life. When emotional events occurred in my life that I had no control over, I subconsciously turned to my eating disorder to give me the sense of control I was lacking. Everyone has his/her coping mechanisms for dealing with unpleasant times; mine was just extremely dangerous and unhealthy.

I've learned now to recognize when I am using food or exercise as a coping mechanism, and I have a number of other, much more helpful and fulfilling ways to deal with the stress that life brings.

Risk Factors

PART FOUR

Special Considerations

I recently noticed that my sister has scars on her arms and wrists. I am concerned that she may be intentionally hurting herself. Why would she do this?

What ethnic groups are affected by anorexia?

What effect does anorexia have on relationships?

More . . .

28. I recently noticed that my sister has scars on her arms and wrists. I am concerned that she may be intentionally hurting herself. Why would she do this?

Certainly, it can be disturbing to know that a loved one may be engaging in this form of behavior. While these behaviors may strike you as being highly unusual and may indeed be quite troubling, you should know that self-injury is becoming increasingly common among eating disorder patients. Approximately 25% of people with an eating disorder engage in self-injurious behaviors. The risk increases with the presence of certain co-occurring mood and personality disorders. Self-injury (also called self-mutilation, self-harm, or self-abuse) is defined in the *Journal of Clinical Psychiatry* as behavior involving the deliberate infliction of physical harm to one's own body without any intent to die as a consequence of that behavior. In other words, self-injury is *not* necessarily an attempt at suicide, although that possibility should always be considered (if your loved one's behavior raises concerns for his or her immediate safety, contact 911 or bring your loved one to a local emergency room for evaluation). Examples of common modes of self-injury include hair-pulling, skin-cutting, head-banging, skin-picking or scratching, biting, hitting, or burning. Often, patients who engage in self-harm may injure themselves on areas of their body that are less visible (such as their shoulders, upper arms, or thighs), or they may try to cover any residual scarring in an attempt to conceal their behavior; however, attempts at secrecy are often unsuccessful.

Approximately 25% of people with an eating disorder engage in self-injurious behaviors.

What motivates a person to self-injure? Usually, and perhaps not surprisingly, patients may self-injure as a means of coping with very uncomfortable emotions. People who self-injure report extreme feelings of tension, anxiety, stress, or emotional pain just before harming themselves. Patients sometimes see self-injury as a way of distracting themselves from that pain or "releasing it" in an attempt to self-soothe; many report that self-injury makes them "numb" to their emotions, bringing them a sensation of peace or temporary relief. Conversely, some patients who self-injure report feeling "dead inside" and "numb" to emotional states. In these cases, self-injury becomes a means of reminding themselves that they are "alive on the inside." Self-harm can also be a form of self-punishment for behaviors that bring shame or guilt. Self-injury is often a vicious cycle, given that the perceived relief is only temporary and does not represent a means for dealing with the underlying issues. In fact, the shame that people feel after harming themselves may lead to additional attempts at self-harm.

The cycle of self-injurious behavior may yield an increased sense of desperation, potentially involving attempts at suicide. Therefore, self-injurious behavior should always be taken seriously. Indeed, studies show that the risk of suicide is a serious and substantial concern for patients with anorexia nervosa. Research indicates that approximately 25% of anorexia-related deaths are due to suicide and that patients with anorexia often use extremely lethal methods when attempting suicide, indicating a strong wish to die. Therefore, anorexia patients should be monitored closely for suicide risk. Factors that may increase the risk of suicide are age at onset of anorexia, longer duration of the illness, lower body weight, certain co-occurring psychiatric disorders, and substance abuse. Additionally, recent studies have suggested that patients who take certain antidepressant medications should be monitored for increased risk of suicidal thinking and suicidal behavior; this is particularly a consideration for children and adolescents.

If your loved one shows signs of self-injury, please encourage them to get help. At the very least, self-injury represents a threat to an individual's overall well-being and quality of life. The reality is that self-injury can cause more harm than intended and can result in serious medical complications, or even death. A healthcare professional can help determine the

Special Considerations

immediacy of risk in your loved one's situation and assess the need for intensive treatment or hospitalization. Remember that self-injurious behavior may be one of the only ways your loved one knows how to cope with their feelings of distress, so try not to judge, blame, or criticize them for their behavior. Express your concern for their well-being, and let them know that you want to help. If you do not feel comfortable talking to them about their self-injuries, be honest about your limits. The important things are to let your loved one know of your concern and to point them toward help and appropriate care.

29. What ethnic groups are affected by anorexia?

Until recently, eating disorders were thought of as illnesses that disproportionately affected Caucasian females. However, several recent studies suggest that the risk for anorexia across ethnic groups may be similar. For example, a recent report published in the *Psychological Bulletin* compiled the results of nearly 100 studies that examined body dissatisfaction among women of different ethnicities. Researchers found that body dissatisfaction was a strong predictor of eating disorders across each of the ethnic groups. Studies report that in the U.S., disordered eating patterns do appear to be equally common among Caucasian and Hispanic females and slightly less common among Black and Asian females (although studies show that the risk among Asian females is increasing), and slightly more common among Native Americans. Other studies indicate that the risk of eating disorders in ethnic minority populations is higher when the degree of **acculturation** is higher. It appears that no ethnic group is immune to the dangers of developing anorexia. Of special concern, however, is that studies in North America indicate ethnic minority women are less likely to be sought out for eating disorders research, less likely to seek care, and less likely to receive treatment for an eating disorder. These findings are disquieting and mark the need for increased efforts at prevention and treatment for underserved populations.

No ethnic group is immune to the dangers of developing anorexia.

Acculturation

Adapting to another culture or modification of one's culture through contact with another culture.

30. I really want to become pregnant, but I'm afraid to because I'm just beginning my journey of recovery. What are some of the effects of pregnancy on women with anorexia?

First, you should know that anorexia and other eating disorders have recently been implicated as a cause of infertility in women of childbearing age. As many as 5–15% of women treated for infertility have a history of eating disorder symptoms, and anorexia patients are particularly susceptible to low rates of fertility. Poor nutrition, endocrine changes caused by low body weight, and excessive exercise can affect fertility. Your doctor will help you determine if your history of anorexia may affect your ability to conceive. However, if you are currently experiencing any symptoms of anorexia, it is better that you continue with your progress in recovery rather than try to enhance fertility when you are underweight or at risk for medical complications. For reasons that will affect both you and your baby, you should wait until you, your doctor, and your treatment team are sure that you are ready to become pregnant.

Issues of fertility aside, pregnancy can be a serious challenge for someone with a history of anorexia and can pose risks to an expectant mother. For example, someone not fully recovered, or not ready for pregnancy, risks a return of eating disorder behaviors, both while pregnant and after giving birth. Therefore, monitoring your symptoms, even if you have been in recovery for some time, is important throughout the duration of your pregnancy as well as postpartum. Some of the potential maternal complications associated with eating disorders include hypertension, vaginal bleeding, cesarean deliveries, anemia, and postpartum depression. In addition, failure to maintain adequate body weight and nutrition during pregnancy can result in the need for hospitalization and intravenous feeding.

Anorexia in an expectant mother can also increase the risk of complications to a developing fetus; complications that can

Special Considerations

affect a child long after birth. Risk of fetal and infant complications include higher rates of miscarriage, infant mortality, premature birth, low birth-weight, low **APGAR** scores, malformations (including cleft lip and palate), respiratory problems, failure to thrive, and delayed development. Abuse of caffeine, diet pills, diuretics, and/or laxatives is particularly dangerous to a fetus. In addition, low maternal weight, purging, and poor nutrition can lead to cognitive, sensory, and physical defects in children. Maternal anorexia is also associated with more disturbed feeding behaviors and a higher rate of depression in children. Mothers with a history of eating disorders may have increased difficulty with breastfeeding and may be excessively concerned with their children's eating behaviors and body weight. For all of these reasons, it is very important that mothers with a history of anorexia receive ongoing collaboration and monitoring from their treatment team throughout the duration of their pregnancy. Mothers should be sure to share their eating disorder symptoms with their gynecologist/obstetrician in order to receive the best prenatal and perinatal care. Additionally, mothers should discuss their infants' food plan with a doctor in order to ensure that their children receive adequate nutrition.

31. I have read that people with anorexia have low self-esteem. Is this true?

Of the personality factors reported among patients with anorexia, poor **self-image** and low **self-esteem** are often an issue. Specifically, many anorexia patients report that they lack a personal sense of self-worth or value and see themselves as "inadequate." Although not everyone with self-esteem concerns develops anorexia, low self-esteem is known to be one of the factors that can serve to increase overall eating disorders risk.

Even healthy individuals commonly report that body shape, weight, and appearance affect the way that they feel about themselves. For individuals with anorexia, however, these factors play an exaggerated role in determining their sense of

APGAR

A test to determine the physical health of a newborn baby. The total score is based on five categories: color, cry, muscle tone, respiration, and reflexes.

Self-image

An individual's perception of his or her own self.

Self-esteem

Personal opinions, judgments, or feelings about oneself.

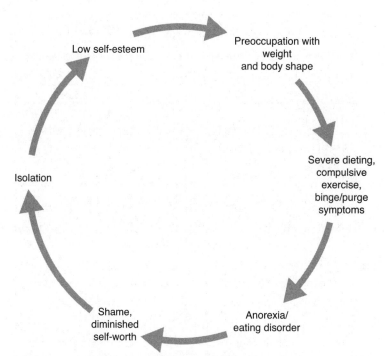

Figure 3   Factors Influencing a Cycle of Low Self-Esteem

self-worth and self-esteem. For the person at risk, restrictive dieting and weight loss may begin as an attempt to compensate for feelings of low self-worth. The pursuit of thinness, then, becomes a means of attaining acceptance from others and increasing personal self-esteem. The body shape and weight pursued by those with anorexia usually represent the quest of an unattainable ideal, an endless pursuit that actually serves to decrease, rather than enhance, self-esteem and self-image. As a result, a cycle of personal shame, self-defeat, and diminished self-worth often ensues (see Figure 3).

Given the link between self-esteem and eating disorder symptoms, recovery from anorexia often includes learning ways of developing a healthier sense of self-worth and personal value. Indeed, expanding self-esteem to include more than just issues of personal appearance is key for any healthy individual, let alone one who has struggled with an eating disorder.

Exhibit 8   Self-Esteem Quick Test

Choose the statement that best describes you. Most of the time do you:

a) Accept compliments?	b) Negate them?
a) Consider the total picture of who you are and what you have accomplished?	b) Look for the blemishes (errors) in the total picture and dwell on them?
a) Like things about your physical self?	b) Look for and point out your own shortcomings?
a) Reach a goal and savor it?	b) Reach a goal and think you should have done better or should have done more?
a) Prefer the company of others?	b) Prefer solitude and isolation?
a) Like your friends and seek them out?	b) Tolerate your friends or try to avoid them?

If you chose all of the answers in the "a" column, you likely have a strong sense of self-esteem and base your self-image on a broad variety of factors. On the other hand, if you chose answers mainly from the "b" column, you may need to spend time strengthening your self-esteem and expand the number and type of qualities you consider when determining your own self-worth.

SOURCE: Adapted from *The Beginner's Guide to Eating Disorders Recovery* by Nancy J. Kolodny. Used with permission.

Exhibit 8 presents a quick test that may help you or a loved one determine if self-esteem issues are of concern.

32. I am a real perfectionist. People tell me I am too "hard on myself," but I just like to do things well. I also have certain ideas about what my body should look like and specific goals about my weight. Will this interfere with my treatment?

Perfectionism refers to the tendency to expect a greater performance from oneself or others than is required for a given situation (Wonderlich 2002). As the term implies, perfectionists set extremely high (and unrealistic) standards for themselves. A growing body of research indicates that perfectionism plays an important role in a number of psychological disorders, including anorexia nervosa. In fact, recent studies suggest that perfectionism is one of the most common traits associated with eating disorders. Studies also suggest that perfectionism is both an **antecedent** risk factor for anorexia and that it appears to persist long after weight recovery from anorexia.

Antecedent
Preceding event or cause.

For some patients, the chronic, telltale traits associated with perfectionism may even indicate a more severe disorder known as obsessive-compulsive personality disorder, or OCPD (see Exhibit 9). Symptoms of OCPD include excessive orderliness, severe inflexibility, extreme stubbornness, and preoccupation with rules and details. Although estimates of **comorbidity** vary greatly (from 3% to 60%), OCPD is one of the personality disorders shown to frequently co-occur with anorexia nervosa (see Question 17). When OCPD co-occurs with anorexia, long-term treatment will address symptoms of both disorders.

Comorbidity
The occurrence of more than one illness, disease, or diagnosable condition at the same time.

Special Considerations

Exhibit 9 Diagnostic Indicators for Obsessive-Compulsive Personality Disorder (OCPD)

OCPD is defined as a pervasive pattern of preoccupation with orderliness, perfectionism, and mental and interpersonal control, at the expense of flexibility, openness, and efficiency, beginning by early adulthood and present in a variety of contexts.

A partial list of associated behaviors may include:

- A preoccupation with details, rules, lists, organization, or schedules
- Perfectionism that interferes with task completion
- Overconscientiousness or inflexibility
- Reluctance to delegate tasks and an inability to work with others unless they submit to an exact way of doing things
- Rigidity and stubbornness

SOURCE: American Psychiatric Association. (1994). *Diagnostic and statistical manual of mental disorders*, 4th ed., Text Revision (p. 729). Washington, DC: Author.

It is one thing to be a high-achiever and to want to give your best effort at essential tasks—this is true of many healthy individuals. However, the self-imposed standard of perfection seen in anorexia patients goes far beyond the adaptive qualities of a conscientious worker or a high achiever. Chronic perfectionism can actually interfere with a healthy attitude about oneself, hinder interpersonal relationships, and negatively affect mental health and well-being. Do any of these characteristics describe your own personality style: inflexible, preoccupied with rules and order, rigid, stubborn, insecure, overly cautious, self-critical, or terrified of making mistakes? Characterized as "neurotic perfectionism," this personality style reflects an "all-or-nothing" mindset that can have a detrimental effect on your quality of life. In fact, instead of increasing self-esteem and a sense of competency, perfectionism often has the opposite effect, increasing feelings of inadequacy, worthlessness, and self-hatred. Perfectionism, therefore, sets a trap: The more it causes you to focus on being the "best" in everything, the more it makes you aware of your shortcomings. Susan Kano, author of *Making Peace with Food,* has this to say about perfectionism: "[While] our search for perfection may sound like a positive thing—like a search for greatness, *in truth a search for perfection is always a search for fault.*" Perfectionism offers a vision of fulfillment and happiness, says Kano, but leaves us with a judgmental inner voice that repeatedly reminds us that we will never be "good enough."

Perfectionism sets a trap: The more it causes you to focus on being the "best" in everything, the more it makes you aware of your shortcomings.

Perfectionism can be especially problematic when it creeps into the area of body image and weight. "*If only* I lose 10 pounds, *then* I will be pretty," "I will be popular *when I lose more weight,*" "I will be happy with myself *only when* I am thinner." These "if only" conditions may seem like commonly expressed sentiments, but for the person at risk for anorexia, thinking of this kind can perpetuate a dangerous cycle of self-disgust, self-deprivation, and unhealthy self-restrictions. Self-imposed restrictions can take on a more dangerous tone: "I cannot eat today until I run 5 *extra miles,*" "I am not good enough unless I am *the thinnest one* of all my friends," "If I eat *anything* today before dinner, I am a failure."

Many people in recovery from anorexia nervosa are also "recovering perfectionists." In such cases, treatment will include attention to changing and adapting one's thinking style so that it is more open, flexible, and self-accepting. In fact, studies show that increasing self-esteem and self-acceptance in treatment assures a better recovery outcome from anorexia. Your therapist and treatment team will help you move away from a place of self-judgment and self-criticism toward a more forgiving and peaceful self-appreciation. It will take time, but the journey toward self-acceptance is well worth the effort. Imagine having a positive outlook about yourself and your life; imagine quieting the "tapes" that play in your mind and seem to highlight your mistakes and faults; imagine feeling valuable and worthy of love. Such an achievement does not have to remain an "*if only*"—it is possible—you *can* learn to feel better about yourself, to accept yourself, and to put an end to the "*if only's.*"

Sarah shares:

One of the hardest parts of my treatment was learning to let go of the unrealistic standards I had set for myself. Even when I did meet my stringent expectations, I convinced myself that it was only because I had set the bar too low; each time I "succeeded" at one of my self-destructive goals, my reward was to make my standards even higher. As you could guess, this mindset quickly deteriorated my mind and body, leaving me with a sense of hopelessness and self-hatred.

In treatment, I discovered that my self-worth is not determined by the calories I restrict or the miles I run. As a "recovering perfectionist," not only did I learn that my weight doesn't establish my self-worth, I realized that the strength of my character is not determined by my grades in school, the number of community service hours I complete, or the amount of money I save. I am not a number, and no quantitative statement can determine my character.

"Should" is a bad word to use when talking about your physical appearance—there is no one way that anyone "should" look, and

I've let go of judging myself based on who the world tries to tell me I "should" be.

33. One thing that I notice about myself is that I have an aversion to sex. This can't be from the anorexia, can it?

This may surprise you, but yes, it can. Remember Ancel Keys and his classic semi-starvation study (see Question 13)? Some of the outcomes noted in this study were the changes that took place in social relationships and sexual desire. With increased calorie restriction and duration of weight-loss, participants became progressively more withdrawn, social contacts with the opposite sex diminished sharply, and interpersonal relationships took on a strained tone. According to accounts, the sexual interests of the volunteers dramatically decreased. Sexual impulses, fantasies, and masturbation either ceased or dramatically diminished. This finding is particularly salient to your question. In fact, it has been suggested that for some adults who have sexual conflicts, dieting and severe food restriction may actually be an attempt to *curtail* sexual concerns and discomfort. According to the *Handbook of Treatment for Eating Disorders*, some adolescent patients may engage in restrictive dieting in the hope of delaying sexual maturity, reducing the appearance of secondary sex characteristics, and diminishing sexual concerns at a time when they feel unprepared to embrace their own sexuality. The presumption is that sexual intimacy can be avoided by making the body less aesthetically appealing and diminishing the appearance of an "adult sexual being."

Heightened body consciousness and body image issues may likewise contribute to increased sexual aversion among eating disorder patients. For patients who experience body image distortion, it can be difficult enough to view their own naked bodies; to be naked with another is unthinkable.

In *Gaining: The Truth about Life after Eating Disorders*, author Aimee Liu, herself a former anorexia patient, states: "among people with eating disorders, the realm of sexuality is particularly fraught." Liu cites two scientific studies that demonstrate that eating disorder patients have lower than normal sexual arousal, desire, and orgasmic functioning, along with increased "sexual discord." Issues of trust, vulnerability, shame, and intimacy are significantly heightened in a sexual relationship or encounter—issues that can be particularly uncomfortable for anorexia patients. As Liu confirms, whether a precursor or an effect of the illness, sexual intimacy is one area of social and emotional functioning that may be dramatically impacted by anorexia nervosa.

34. My daughter has been recovered for a couple of years and is doing well. I am concerned because she has made friends with a couple girls who look really underweight and unhealthy. Should I worry that her friendships could lead to a relapse?

This can be a difficult question to answer. On the one hand, peer weight-loss behaviors and dietary restriction among close friends have been shown to influence adolescent attitudes about food and weight. If a teen wants to feel "part of the crowd" or be accepted by a group of peers who emphasize thinness, it can be difficult to go against the tide of peer attitudes. Social peers who engage in eating disorder behaviors such as calorie restriction and purging can be a source of vulnerability for someone at risk. On the other hand, research also shows that supportive friendships can both protect teens from developing an eating disorder and may help in recovery from an existing eating disorder.

You may want to speak with your daughter in a gentle, nonthreatening way that does not accuse her friends, but instead encourages open and honest communication. You will want to know if your daughter notices any high-risk behaviors or harmful attitudes toward food, weight, and body shape in her friends. Ask her if their behaviors have been discussed among the group. Perhaps her friends are in treatment themselves; if so they may be a source of support for your daughter and friends with whom she feels comfortable sharing her own experiences of recovery. If they are not in treatment, or if they appear to be encouraging eating disordered behavior, you may want to consider limiting the amount of contact she has with them. However, you should approach this matter very carefully with your daughter, as a teen's friendships can be an extremely important and influential source of support. Be careful to not attack her friends, judge them, or put them down in any way. Instead, communicate your reasons for concern.

Also, consider speaking with her in private, not when her friends are present. You will want to ensure there are other avenues for support in your child's life to prevent feelings of isolation, peer rejection, and resentment, all of which can trigger eating disorder symptoms. It may be helpful to suggest that your daughter discuss this matter with her treatment team for additional support. Lastly, you may want to communicate to your daughter that you will remain open to discussing this matter with her periodically, amending the need for limited contact with this group should the situation change.

35. I think I may have an eating disorder, but I'm not ready to get help for it. I don't want my family to be concerned, so I'm hiding my weight loss from them. I also usually eat alone and hide how much I exercise from them. I don't know how much longer I can keep this up. What should I do?

It is not unusual for someone with anorexia to live certain aspects of their lives in secret.

Hiding behaviors associated with anorexia is quite common. It is not unusual for someone with anorexia to live certain aspects of their lives in secret, eating alone, weighing themselves when no one is looking, purging in secret. Individuals may also lie to loved ones about their behavior (e.g., "I'm just not hungry because I ate a big lunch," or, "This outfit just makes me look thin."); however, the reality is that lying about your illness and hiding your eating disorder is only cheating yourself.

One reason you may feel "protective" of your eating disorder is that unlike with other mental illnesses, such as depression or anxiety, the symptoms of anorexia are "ego-syntonic," a technical term that means the behaviors and feelings associated with anorexia are often welcome and acceptable to patients, rather than distressing and uncomfortable. Indeed, many anorexia patients reportedly experience certain "benefits" from their illness. A 2002 issue of the *European Eating Disorders Review* recorded some of these perceived benefits, as expressed by patients in recovery. Responses included:

- "Anorexia gives me a sense of control."
- "Anorexia is my way of avoiding serious problems."
- "Anorexia is my way of escaping thoughts about myself that I do not like."
- "Anorexia distracts me from my painful emotions."
- "Anorexia allows me to avoid my fears about sex and sexuality."
- "Anorexia makes me feel unique and special."

Feelings such as these serve to reinforce anorexic behaviors and cause patients to feel stuck. They may know anorexia is not good for them, but they do not know what else to do. The writers of *Anorexia Nervosa: A Guide to Recovery* put it this way: "Anorexia is a paradox, because while it is slowly killing you, it is also serving you in some way. It is natural to fear the uncertainty of what life would be like without it."

Eating disorders are dangerously insidious. Although you may not feel ready to tell your family, please consider telling *someone*. Your doctor, therapist, teacher, school nurse, a trusted friend (another person who is not struggling with an eating disorder themselves). If you are able to tell even one trusted person who is concerned for your health and safety, you can reduce the sense of living in secret and isolation—and you may then feel more ready to receive help. It is far better to take steps to arm yourself against the devastating consequences of this illness than to let it have the upper hand. Please, don't be silent any longer. Tell a trusted loved one what you are going through.

Lynn shares:

For over a decade, I believed that I hid my eating disorder from family and friends. Most people close to you actually know more than you think about what is going on, but they don't know what to do or how to help, which is even more stressful for them. There was a lot of denial involved for me. I believed I knew what I was doing and that I knew better than friends, family, coaches, and doctors. I had national records in races to confirm this in my mind. As the disease progressed, I could feel and sense the dangers, yet the fear of losing control and the fear of gaining weight were as strong (often stronger) than the fear of dying. The longer I stayed in the disorder, the harder it was to get out. Ironically, the more I wanted to feel in control by staying in the anorexia, the more the anorexia controlled me. When I finally did try to get help, I discovered that no one could "control me" out of the disorder. No one can ever force you in the long run to eat and gain weight. I would always have the choice to stay in the eating disorder and allow it to control me and even kill me. Recovery was much different than I expected. In recovery I truly did learn how to take control of my own life, and the world then seemed to open up to me in ways I never imagined.

Sarah shares:

For a long time I tried to hide my strange behaviors from friends and family. I told everyone at school that I had an overactive thyroid gland and that I just ran for fun. But despite my attempts to be sly, I don't think anyone was fooled by my act. I let my eating disorder get to the point where there was no more hiding it, and even then, letting go of anorexia was one of the scariest things imaginable.

An eating disorder is not just a made-up sickness that you can cure on your own, and as terrifying as it might seem to let go of your eating disorder and live a normal life, it is SO much scarier to let it get the best of you. My parents had to literally drag me to the door of my treatment center, and though I never thought I would say it, going to treatment was the best thing that has ever happened to me.

36. What effect does anorexia have on relationships?

Anorexia nervosa is an isolating illness. The mood and personality changes that result from semi-starvation can wreak havoc on close personal relationships and family ties. To begin with, the symptoms of anorexia demand a great deal of focus and attention: calorie counting, meal planning, exercise, purging behaviors, preoccupation with weight, and scrutinizing of one's own appearance and body image. All of these require energy, which is already a limited commodity for the person in a semi-starved state. Thus, anorexia patients often gradually restrict their activities and narrow their interests to those having to do with food restriction, exercise, and necessary work or schoolwork.

Anorexia can take its toll on close relationships. For many loved ones, feelings of powerlessness, frustration, and resentment can build, increasing strain and inadvertently furthering the pattern of patient isolation and withdrawal. Fear and discomfort at the sight of an emaciated loved one can make for understandably tense interactions. Indeed, some recoil out of a paralyzing uncertainty about "what to say" (e.g., "Should I tell her that she looks frail?" "Do I treat her as though there is nothing wrong?"). Irritability and moodiness, constant fighting over meals, tense outings at the supermarket, desperate attempts to get a loved one to eat; all of these patterns can result in guilt, anxiety, worry, resentment, and anger, emotions that can strain family and marital relationships. Sadly, anorexia has been known to destroy the connectedness that was once shared in otherwise loving families.

Relationship problems may be further compounded in social gatherings that center on food due to the enormous pressure

Exhibit 10   Diagnostic Indicators for Avoidant Personality Disorder (AVPD)

AVPD is defined as a pervasive pattern of social inhibition, marked by feelings of inadequacy and hypersensitivity to negative evaluation, beginning by early adulthood and present in a variety of contexts, as indicated by four (or more) of the following:

- Avoids occupational activities that involve significant interpersonal contact because of fears of criticism, disapproval, or rejection.
- Is unwilling to get involved with people unless certain of being liked.
- Shows restraint within intimate relationships because of the fear of being shamed or ridiculed.
- Is preoccupied with being criticized or rejected in social situations.
- Is inhibited in new interpersonal situations because of feelings of inadequacy.
- Views self as socially inept, personally unappealing, or inferior to others.
- Is unusually reluctant to take personal risks or to engage in any new activities because they may prove embarrassing.

SOURCE: American Psychiatric Association. (1994). *Diagnostic and statistical manual of mental disorders*, 4th ed., Text Revision (p. 721). Washington, DC: Author.

anorexia patients experience in such situations. Some patients will eat socially but only to keep up appearances while they simultaneously experience an overwhelming urge to restrict. Others face frantic feelings of anxiety and are distracted by the need to purge or compensate for calories ingested. Social discomfort is further exacerbated when there is co-occurring social phobia, a social anxiety disorder often found in anorexia patients. Such individuals may *desire* interpersonal connectedness but avoid social situations due to intense fear or anxiety.

Two related disorders that frequently co-occur in patients with anorexia are avoidant personality disorder (AVPD) and dependent personality disorder (DPD) (see Exhibits 10 and 11). In AVPD, people display pervasive and long-standing traits of shyness, social withdrawal, stranger anxiety, and

> **Exhibit 11   Diagnostic Indicators for Dependent Personality Disorder (DPD)**
>
> DPD is defined as a pervasive and excessive need to be taken care of that leads to submissive, clinging behavior and fears of separation, beginning by early adulthood and present in a variety of contexts. A partial list of associated behaviors may include:
>
> - Difficulty making everyday decisions without an excessive amount of advice and reassurance from others.
> - Need for others to assume responsibility for most major areas of his or her life.
> - Difficulty expressing disagreement with others because of fear of loss of support or approval.
> - Difficulty initiating projects or doing things on one's own.
> - Going to excessive lengths to obtain nurturance and support from others.
> - Feeling uncomfortable or helpless when alone and urgently seeking another relationship as a source of support when a close relationship ends.
> - Unrealistic fears of being left to take care of himself or herself.
>
> SOURCE: American Psychiatric Association. (1994). *Diagnostic and statistical manual of mental disorders*, 4th ed., Text Revision (p. 721). Washington, DC: Author.

fearfulness in social situations. Individuals with AVPD generally have a negative self-evaluation, feel socially "incompetent," and are therefore quite reluctant to become involved in activities that require social interaction. An estimated 15–25% of eating disorder patients with a co-occurring personality disorder are diagnosed with AVPD. In contrast, patients with DPD are described as "extreme people pleasers." These individuals tend to intensely fear separation from others, excessively seek reassurance or caretaking from loved ones, and have difficulty asserting their own opinions or desires. Individuals with DPD are often terrified of losing approval or support; therefore, they are often reluctant to disagree with others. Anorexia patients who are already prone to self-doubt and self-criticism belittle their own abilities to an even greater degree when DPD is present.

Lynn shares:

I was entrenched in my eating disorder throughout my teen and young adult years, which is the time that most people go through puberty and learn much about successful relationships. I always believed I had no problems with relationships. In one way it was true, because I didn't have any real relationships. I was focused almost entirely on the eating disorder for a couple of decades. After achieving some recovery, I struggled in my first job because I didn't have good relationship skills. I was one of the hardest working and dedicated employees, but I never let anyone know who I was. Most people are very uncomfortable with this. It was a team environment, and I didn't know how to be a team member. I couldn't be invisible any longer. I finally understood how the many years in the eating disorder had kept me from learning basic social interactions, especially those derived from a real sense of self-confidence, which is vital for survival in the business world.

Sarah shares:

My eating disorder consumed every moment of every day and became the only steady relationship in my life. It prevented me from ever keeping a boyfriend or making new friends, and after a while, even my closest friends gave up on me. I distinctly remember one time when my two best friends came over to my house simply to tell me, "We give up. We just can't do this anymore, Sarah." That was when I completely lost hope. If even my best friends didn't believe I could overcome my anorexia, how could I believe in myself?

At the worst of it, everything I did was dictated by a voice inside my head that made me feel like the only means of being in control of my life were running more, eating less, and essentially destroying my body. In reality, it was quite the opposite: The more I let my anorexia control me, the less control I had over my life.

PART FIVE

Exercise and Athletes

How much exercise is "too much" exercise?

Are athletes at greater risk for developing anorexia and eating disorders?

What is the "female athlete triad"?

More . . .

37. How much exercise is "too much" exercise?

There are no specific, global standards for judging whether exercise behavior is excessive; therefore, what may be appropriate levels of exercise for one person may be unhealthy levels of exercise for another. There are, however, methods for assessing "exercise dependence." Recommended guidelines for *healthy* exercise generally include activity that occurs 3–6 days per week for approximately 30–60 minutes per day. However, even moderate exercise can be excessive for a patient weakened by anorexia and malnutrition, so anorexia patients should discuss with their doctor if exercise is appropriate. Exercising in a weakened physical state can be extremely dangerous and can lead to electrolyte imbalances, heart arrhythmias, and other serious medical complications.

Here are some questions to ask yourself to help determine if you are exercising excessively:

- Are you exercising more than 5 days a week for more than 1 hour per day?
- Are you exercising more than your coach, doctor, or parents recommend?
- Do you exercise in order to lose weight because you feel obligated to, or because you enjoy the activity?
- Do you try to squeeze in "hidden" exercise (e.g., running an extra flight of stairs or doing extra jumping jacks) in order to compensate for calories consumed?
- Do you take care to increase the amount of calories consumed in order to fuel your body for physical activity? Emily Cooper, medical director and founder of Seattle Performance Medicine gives this helpful tip to her patients: *"If you can't fuel it, don't do it!"*
- Does the amount of time you spend exercising interfere with other important areas of your life?
- Do you exercise when you are injured or ill?

Healthy exercise tends to be social and enjoyable and is engaged in irrespective of the amount of food eaten. In contrast, unhealthy, excessive exercise tends to be obligatory, performed in isolation, and is undertaken with the primary goal of losing weight or burning off calories that have been ingested. Exercise that is excessive or interferes with physical or emotional health may be an indicator of something known as *exercise dependence*.

Exercise Dependence

The term exercise dependence (also known as "compulsive exercise" or "exercise addiction") describes physical exercise that is excessive in frequency, duration, or intensity. It is characterized as a craving for physical activity that results in extreme exercise and generates negative physiological symptoms (such as injury) and negative psychological symptoms (such as guilt, depression, irritability, restlessness, tension, anxiety, and sluggishness) (Hausenblas and Symons Downs 2002). According to the *DSM-IV-TR*, exercise becomes excessive when it significantly interferes with important activities, when it occurs at inappropriate times or in inappropriate settings, or when a person continues exercising despite an injury or other medical complication.

Researchers at the University of Florida and Pennsylvania State University developed a useful measure to assess for exercise dependence (see Exhibit 12). It evaluates seven different aspects of exercise dependence, including tolerance, **withdrawal** effects, continuance of exercise despite injury or other physical problems, lack of control, reduction of other activities (e.g., spending time with family or friends), time spent exercising, and intention (e.g., exercising for longer than was planned). Treatment teams may use a measure such as this in order to determine if one's level of exercise meets the criteria for exercise dependence.

Withdrawal

Characteristic symptoms that occur after the cessation of long-term use, or the sudden discontinuation of a drug or habit-forming action.

Exercise and Athletes

Exhibit 12   Exercise Dependence Scale-21

Instructions: Using the scale provided, please complete the following questions as honestly as possible. The questions refer to current exercise beliefs and behaviors that have occurred in the past 3 months. Please place your answer in the blank space provided after each statement.

1	2	3	4	5	6
Never					Always

1. I exercise to avoid feeling irritable._____
2. I exercise despite recurring physical problems._____
3. I continually increase my exercise intensity to achieve the desired effects/benefits._____
4. I am unable to reduce how long I exercise._____
5. I would rather exercise than spend time with family/friends._____
6. I spend a lot of time exercising._____
7. I exercise longer than I intend._____
8. I exercise to avoid feeling anxious._____
9. I exercise when injured._____
10. I continually increase my exercise frequency to achieve the desired effects/benefits._____
11. I am unable to reduce how often I exercise._____
12. I think about exercise when I should be concentrating on school/work._____
13. I spend most of my free time exercising._____
14. I exercise longer than I expect._____
15. I exercise to avoid feeling tense._____
16. I exercise despite persistent physical problems._____
17. I continually increase my exercise duration to achieve the desired effects/benefits._____
18. I am unable to reduce how intensely I exercise._____
19. I choose to exercise so that I can get out of spending time with family/friends._____
20. A great deal of my time is spent exercising._____
21. I exercise longer than I plan._____

SOURCES: Hausenblas, H. A., and Symons Downs, D. (2002). How much is too much? The development and validation of the Exercise Dependence Scale. *Psychology & Health 17*:387–404. Used with permission.

Symons Downs, D., Hausenblas, H. A., & Nigg, C. R. (2004). Factorial validity and psychometric examination of the Exercise Dependence Scale-Revised. *Measurement in Physical Education and Exercise Science 8*:183–201. Used with permission.

When a Child or Teen Is Overexercising

When it comes to excessive exercise, knowing when to intervene and what steps to take can be complicated. Parents should consult their family physician to determine if their child is within a healthy weight range for his or her level of physical activity. If he or she is underweight or shows signs of an eating disorder, your doctor may recommend placing limits on duration and intensity of exercise permitted (e.g., a physician may recommend "rest days" of inactivity). The challenge for parents is to enforce any recommended restrictions. It may be especially difficult if exercise has been a source of pleasure and mastery for a teen athlete. Be firm in your enforcing of limits, knowing that it is in your child's best health interests. Try to include your child in the discussion, rather than imposing restrictions in a way that hinders open communication. If your child is part of a team sport, you may consider allowing continued attendance at team events so your child can maintain a connection to the team. A note of interest: You may be surprised at the outcome of your intervention. Some teens report feeling *relieved* when they are encouraged to reduce their exercise intensity, and others report discovering talents, strengths, and abilities of which they were previously unaware.

Even if a child is within the normal weight range, excessive exercise itself can be harmful. Be sure that the child's physician approves any exercise routine and that he is not involved in more activity than his coach or trainer recommends. Parents may also need to contact a child's coach and/or physical education teacher to ensure that they have a flexible approach to training and to elicit their support in monitoring compliance with physician recommendations. Keep in mind that when recommended, abstaining from exercise is usually only a temporary restriction; when a physician gives approval, parents can begin to loosen any exercise restrictions that have been set in place. Often, parents find it best to allow some mild activity to be reinstated as incremental treatment goals are met; however, this varies case by case. Finally, parents should stay in contact with their family physician and report any noncompliance with treatment recommendations and exercise restrictions. Studies show that noncompliance with exercise restrictions may be an indicator of an eating disorder or risk for relapse.

A Healthy Example at Home

A balanced approach to diet and exercise in the home can go a long way toward developing healthy attitudes in kids and teens. Here are some general guidelines to keep in mind:

- Do a self-check on your own attitudes about exercise and physical fitness. Parents who themselves exercise excessively may unintentionally influence their children to follow similar exercise patterns. A balanced, healthy approach is best.
- If your child is an athlete, be sure not to put too much pressure on him or her to excel in sports. It can be damaging when a parent's goal for their child's level of physical activity is unrealistic or motivated by the parent's need to see their child be a "successful athlete." Be supportive of your child's interests but not in a way that might encourage excessive exercise. Also, if you suspect that a coach or physical education teacher is putting undue pressure on your child to excel in athletics, speak to the coach and express your concerns.
- Parents, as well as other significant role models (e.g., coaches, siblings), should be careful not to make critical comments concerning appearance, weight, or body-type that may lead to excessive exercise or diet behaviors.
- Do not mistake apparent high levels of energy for good health. Malnourished patients may seem "fidgety" or appear to have a great deal of energy for athletic activity. Over-activity and restlessness is common with anorexia. In fact, activity level may *increase* as patients continue to lose weight.

Over-activity and restlessness is common with anorexia.

- Speak with your child about the dangers of overexercising. Anorexia patients are especially prone to bone fractures and other health complications. Instead of building muscle, too much exercise can actually damage muscles and can put undue stress on heart function, especially if the body is not getting enough nutrients.
- Know your child's physical limitations.

Lynn shares:

I never had an outside perspective to moderate my excessive exercise tendencies. There was likely a place for moderate exercise during recovery in my case, but it was a long time before I learned how to do "moderate." As a consequence, I dealt with constant injuries that slowed the healing process and the potential return to my sport.

In recovery, I had to ask myself why I was running so hard that day or what I was running from. Early on it is hard to give yourself an honest answer. The goals of the exercise get mixed up in the goals of the disease, and they may be almost impossible to distinguish. Here is where some outside perspective can be most valuable. It is like recovering from an injury. You may need some time for healing before getting back to your athletic goals. Often athletic performance is a way to feel good about yourself, but it doesn't work if that sense of self-esteem is not already in place. Taking some time off to heal body, mind, and soul may be just what it takes to restore your athletic pursuits. Without this healing, and if you remain in the disease, it will likely end those pursuits prematurely—as it did for me—and the resulting long-term consequences can plague you into your older years. When you do return, you may find that you have a whole new perspective and enjoyment of your sport and the freedom to reach for your goals apart from the controlling obsessions of the disease. The enjoyment and lifetime potential in recovery are far beyond what you had before in anorexia.

38. How is exercise approached in the treatment of anorexia nervosa?

Restoration of normal weight is a key aspect of recovery from anorexia nervosa. Studies show that patients who remain underweight are at a greater risk for relapse and for complications. Thus, patients are often restricted from exercising until a normal weight has been achieved. In some cases, the duration of inactivity may be considerable. Generally, the caloric and nutritional needs of a patient with acute anorexia are so great that it is very difficult to sustain weight gain if the patient is engaging in even moderate exercise. When medically necessary, patients who are unable to comply with exercise restrictions may need to be hospitalized to ensure healthy weight restoration. Often exercise can be resumed, in increasing levels of duration and intensity, as established goals of weight restoration and physical health are achieved.

While some studies indicate exercise should be avoided until weight gain is achieved, eating disorder specialists note various approaches to exercise and weight restoration. For example, some suggest that when exercise is well regulated, it may in fact contribute to the recovery process. Those with this viewpoint suggest that a supervised exercise program, such as those frequently provided in residential treatment centers, allows for the mental and physical benefits of activity to contribute to a patient's feelings of normalcy, independence, and social pleasure. In these instances, care is taken to model a balanced approach to physical activity such that moderate exercise is seen as one aspect of a healthy lifestyle. In addition, physical activity may be used in treatment as a means of reinforcing weight gain. For example, a patient who desires to reengage in physical activity may be permitted to do so as a "reward" for achieving a moderate goal of weight restoration. Treatment centers and treating professionals may vary in their approach to the role of exercise in recovery, but in every case, decisions need to be made that are in the best interests of the health and well-being of each individual. A medical doctor should always be consulted when considering the introduction of exercise into the recovery process, and a dietitian should be consulted to ensure adequate dietary and nutritional support.

For patients with the added diagnosis of exercise dependence, a treatment team may suggest some changes in the *pattern* of exercise. For example, changing the order of activities, changing the type of activity (e.g., swimming instead of jogging), or changing the location of an activity may in fact decrease some of the exercise compulsions experienced by a patient. "Changing it up" in an exercise routine may seem simple, but even simple changes can influence a rigid pattern of over-exercise. In addition, exercise dependent patients may need assistance in developing alternative methods for coping with stress and anxiety.

Sarah shares:

Going into treatment, I was afraid that I would never be able to exercise again and that I would turn into an out-of-shape blob with atrophying muscles and no sense of self-control. In fact, things turned out to be quite the opposite. My treatment team never ruled out exercise as an option; they just taught me how to exercise for the right reasons.

I've always been a runner, but instead of running to fulfill a persistent compulsion, I've learned to run because I truly enjoy the way it makes me feel. In 2006, I came in 8th place in my age division at the Freescale Austin Marathon, and when I was done, I didn't give a second thought to the number of calories I had burned. The feeling of accomplishment I get from running now is so much different than it used to be. Instead of running away from things I didn't want to face, now I can run with an end in mind and achieve entirely different goals.

39. *Are athletes at greater risk for developing anorexia and eating disorders?*

Focus, determination, competitive drive, dedication, these are some of the coveted qualities associated with athletes who excel at the highest level of competitive sports. It is these very qualities, however, that may also put some athletes at greater risk for developing an eating disorder. While some evidence suggests that sports and sport participation can provide general benefits to one's overall mental and physical health, experts note certain caveats that apply to various competitive sports and sport environments.

Meta-analysis

A method of analysis that combines the results of a number of scientific studies, each addressing a related research hypothesis.

According to a **meta-analysis** published in a 2000 issue of the *International Journal of Eating Disorders,* sport participation may protect some athletes from eating problems, however, it may *contribute* to an increased risk of such problems for others. Specifically, studies show that athletes who compete in sports in which there is an emphasis on thinness are at greater risk for engaging in unhealthy weight control measures. Performance sports such as dance, cheerleading, gymnastics, swimming, diving, and figure skating are associated with higher rates of eating disorders than other sports. Similarly, athletes who engage in certain elite sports (such as wrestling, jockeying, weight lifting, rowing, cross-country skiing, and long-distance running) and athletes who compete at national or professional levels are also at higher risk.

Estimates of risk for anorexia and other eating disorders among athletes vary, but the numbers are sobering. Studies show that at least one-third of college-aged female athletes demonstrate disordered eating behavior. The American College of Sports Medicine found that eating disorders affect up to 62% of females in such sports as gymnastics and figure skating. Additional findings suggest that female, adolescent ballet dancers are eight times more likely to develop an eating disorder than their non-dieting peers. The prevalence of clinical eating disorders among male athletes appears to be lower than among females, however, experts caution that such cases may go overlooked or underreported.

According to the *Handbook of Eating Disorders*, eating disorders risk increases when athletes (or coaches) "lose contact with what is normal" with regard to healthy eating behaviors, due to the intensity of training for competitive athletics. Failure to achieve the desired weight for athletic performance can be a powerful trigger for unhealthy dieting behaviors and eating disorders. Furthermore, in some athletic subcultures, disordered eating may even be regarded as a natural part of being an athlete. Wrestlers, for example, are often expected to compete in weight classes below their usual body weight, and significant numbers use harmful practices such as restrictive eating, vomiting, laxatives, and diuretics to meet performance goals. In sports such as gymnastics or figure skating, where the athletes are judged by both technical and artistic merit, pressure for thinness increases if it is believed that judges will take body shape into consideration when awarding artistic scores. Along that line, experts note that in 1972, the winning female gymnastics team had an average height of 5′ 3″ and an average weight of 106 pounds, while in 1992, the average height was 4′9″ and the average weight was 83 pounds. Part of this trend in body size among gymnasts has been attributed to a "thin aesthetic." Tragically, one of the world's top gymnasts, Christy Henrich, after being told by a U.S. judge at a 1988 competition in Budapest that she needed to lose weight if she hoped to make the Olympic team, developed bulimia and anorexia. Christy's eating disorder took her life in 1994.

Keeping the risks in mind, it should be noted that athletic participation can be a valuable activity that provides many benefits to general health. Indeed, studies show that for people whose physicians have determined they are healthy enough for regular exercise, athletic participation can contribute to higher levels of self-esteem, lower levels of body dissatisfaction, and fewer symptoms of depression. If you or a loved one are a competitive athlete, be aware of the eating disorders risk factors that have been identified by researchers. These include: over involvement in sports, perfectionism, extreme compliance, obsessive-compulsive tendencies, training when sick or injured, pressure from coaches or parents to lose weight, and changes in coaching personnel. Be sure to weigh the risks and benefits of athletic participation accordingly, and seek consultation with a physician if you are concerned about eating disorders risk. For more information about athletes and eating disorders, a recommended resource is "The BodySense Program" (*www. bodysense.ca*), an initiative of the Canadian Centre for Ethics in Sport that promotes positive body image.

40. I thought lower body fat percentage makes you a better athlete, but now I know this is not true. What are some other misconceptions about weight and sports performance?

Athletes and athletic communities may indeed be misinformed about various issues related to athletic performance and health. In the following list, each bolded statement represents a misconception or myth surrounding nutrition, body weight, and sports performance.

- *The leaner you are, the better athlete you will be.* While a drop in weight may initially increase performance speed in sports, persistent lack of nutrition depletes the body's support system, resulting in decreased performance.
- *Being thinner than your competition means you will perform better than they will.* Research has not shown strong support for the notion that thinness can enhance athletic performance. Sports nutrition and eating disorders researcher Dr. Pauline Powers identifies three more important keys to athletic performance: genetics, muscle mass, and motivation. Comparing competitors by weight may increase the likelihood of unhealthy diet behaviors.

- *Losing your period is normal when you are a female athlete.* Amenorrhea is a sign of insufficient nutrition, hormone imbalance, or lack of adequate body fat. It is *not* normal for healthy development and increases the risk of bone fractures, osteopenia, and early osteoporosis, even among athletes.
- *If an athlete is performing well, he or she must be healthy.* Not necessarily. According to the *Clinical Manual of Eating Disorders,* athletes with symptoms of disordered eating are often able to perform well for some time. However, many of the most serious physiological complications emerge silently and without warning.
- *Taking time off for treatment will interfere with sports performance.* Returning to good health will likely *improve* sports performance. Sports may be an important part of an athlete's life, however, good health is not only a key to sports performance but to overall quality of life.
- *If a coach says an athlete has to lose more weight, it must be the right thing to do.* Coaches can be a great source of support and motivation. However, decisions that affect medical health should be made by, or at least in consultation with, a physician. Well-meaning coaches may put undue pressure on an athlete by making comments about weight and may indeed be misinformed about the relationship between body weight and sports performance.
- *Weight-bearing activities actually reduce the risk for osteoporosis, so an athlete is protected.* Exercise alone does not protect against osteoporosis. Adequate nutrition and a healthy body weight curtail the risk of amenorrhea, which can dramatically increase the risk of osteoporosis.
- *Daily training is necessary to maintain athletic performance.* Actually, muscles need days without exercise to refuel and recover. Taking a day or two off from training does not decrease performance and may in fact have performance benefits.

Exercise and Athletes

41. What is the "female athlete triad"?

The female athlete triad (or "the Triad") is a term that identifies three interrelated problems of female athletes: disordered eating, amenorrhea, and osteoporosis. According to a report published by the Medical Commission of the International Olympic Committee (IOMC), although any one of these problems can occur in isolation, inadequate nutrition in a female athlete may lead to all three occurring in sequence—hence the term "female athlete triad." The IOMC stresses that presence of any one of these components indicates the need to evaluate an athlete for the other two concerns. Furthermore, not all three of these features need be present to warrant concern.

Those at greatest risk for developing the Triad are women who participate in aesthetic sports (e.g., gymnastics, diving, cheerleading) and endurance sports (e.g., swimming, rowing, running), and "weight-class" sports (e.g., body building, karate). Women who are already underweight when they begin sports training are at the greatest risk. Although the occurrence of the Triad is highest in elite athletes, it can occur at any age or athletic skill level. A history of amenorrhea is one of the easiest ways to detect the female athlete triad in its earliest stages. Other menstrual disorders, low energy levels, and low bone mineral density may also serve as early warning signs of the Triad.

Lynn shares:

Many of the elite female distance runners that I met in the 1970s experienced some aspect of the Triad. The absence of a period was only discussed confidentially, and we believed it was due to hard effort rather than low body fat. None of us understood the long-term consequences. Although most would not have been diagnosed with clinical anorexia, many were obsessive about trying to maintain a very low body weight, believing it was essential for optimum performance. I remember being at an international competition in Europe where three of the top women distance runners in the world discussed how fat and inadequate they felt.

The consequences of those years of food and weight obsession, even without a true clinical eating disorder, can chase you into your older years with osteoporosis, stress fractures, injuries, and often continuing obsession with food, weight, and body image. These may not be life threatening or seem severe enough to require a treatment program, but they can decrease quality of life. It is so important and so worthwhile to address these issues early on, when they are easier to treat and the long-term consequences can be lessened.

42. How can coaches be involved in screening for and preventing eating disorders?

First, coaches should be aware of the risk for anorexia and other eating disorders in athletes and learn about warning signs associated with these conditions. Coaches should also learn to recognize when healthy training routines may turn into dangerous obsessions and be willing to consult with healthcare professionals when necessary. Training staff also need to reassure their athletes that they will not be criticized when coming forward for help.

Coaches should strongly consider becoming involved in an athlete's eating disorder recovery process, recognizing that their support and influence may be just as significant as that of a family member. Indeed, athletes care tremendously about the opinions of their coaches, value their input, and will often look to them for advice and support. Coaches therefore have the unique opportunity to present a balanced approach to training, health, and nutrition that will have lasting effects on their athletes. For this reason, coaches are strongly encouraged not to comment on body shape or size, or to require weight loss in young athletes whose bodies are still developing. Coaches should also examine their own beliefs regarding weight, dieting, and sports performance, as these beliefs may inadvertently affect their athletes. Additionally, public weigh-ins should be discouraged or avoided, thus diminishing the risk of increased body-image discomfort or comparisons between athletes.

Exercise and Athletes

Early intervention and prevention strategies should be a priority for coaching staff. The NCAA stresses the need for coaches' involvement in such programs for them to be successful. A program to consider, for example, may include soliciting the help of a nutrition expert to educate athletes about healthy eating, the nutritional needs of athletes in training, the expected increases in weight and body fat in athletes during puberty, and related topics. Another good way for sports programs to get started is to have prepared health and nutrition guidelines and materials that they can make available to all of their athletes. Toward that end, the NCAA has recently published a handbook for coaches about eating disorders and the female athlete triad. In educating themselves, coaches can simultaneously educate their athletes. Additional prevention strategies for coaches are recommended for consideration by the Rader Institute. They include:

- Educating athletes on the symptoms and warning signs of an eating disorder
- Educating athletes on the physical risks of maintaining a low body weight
- Not overplaying the impact of weight on athletic performance
- Promoting healthy nutrition
- Eliminating public weigh-ins
- Providing a resource for emotional counseling
- Eliminating critical remarks about body shape or weight
- Setting realistic goals, taking into account the individual athlete's body type and shape
- Recognizing when healthy training regimens turn into obsessions
- Encouraging positive self-image and self-esteem

PART SIX

Body Image Concerns

What is body image?

What is Body Dysmorphic Disorder?

What are some practical ways to improve body image?

More . . .

43. *What is body image?*

Body image is made up of three core elements: (1) the way you see yourself when you look in the mirror, (2) the mental picture you have of your body, and (3) your attitudes about your body (including your perceptions, feelings, and beliefs). Body image is based in part on the body's actual appearance, but it can also be affected by personal experiences, feelings, and ideas, as well as by interactions with (and reactions from) other people. Beliefs about personal body image affect not only what we believe *about* our bodies; they can also affect the way we feel *in* our bodies. Our own beliefs about our bodies can also affect how we think *other* people perceive our bodies. For example, if you are satisfied with your own appearance and body image, you are more likely to believe other people perceive your body in a positive way, and, conversely, if you are dissatisfied with your own body image and appearance, you are more likely to think others will be dissatisfied with it too.

Positive and Negative Body Image

The terms "positive body image" and "negative body image" describe a person's comfort level with their own body. Positive body image (also called healthy body image or body image acceptance) is generally comprised of a sense of acceptance, comfort, and positive regard for one's own body. In addition, positive body image results from accurate perceptions of one's own appearance. Indeed, people with positive body image are unlikely to think to themselves, "I just *love my body!*" On the contrary, they tend to recognize their own flaws (because, after all, *"no body"* is perfect!). In addition, they are more likely to appreciate their natural body for the benefits it offers. They also generally feel comfortable about their bodies because they understand that their physical body is just *one* part of who they are. Therefore, they are more likely to appreciate their own unique strengths, talents, abilities, and personality. A person with a positive body image spends less time worrying about appearance and therefore has more time to spend in other activities that help build confidence and self-esteem.

Positive body image is generally comprised of a sense of acceptance, comfort, and positive regard for one's own body.

In contrast, negative body image (also called unhealthy body image, body image dissatisfaction, or body image disturbance) is characterized by a sense of shame, embarrassment, disappointment, or even disgust at one's own body. Disapproving thoughts, discomfort, and anxiety often go hand-in-hand with negative body image. People with negative body image are also more likely to focus on the *parts* of their bodies with which they are dissatisfied. The effect of body image disturbance can be far reaching. For example, studies show that greater degrees of body dissatisfaction are associated with poor self-esteem, depression, anxiety, unhealthy dieting behaviors, and eating disorders. Poor body image can affect one's mood, social functioning, and even level of sexual fulfillment. In contrast to those with a healthy body image, people with a negative body image are less likely to give themselves praise for other strengths and personality characteristics. This is because they are more likely to ascribe their sense of value or worth to their appearance and/or body shape.

For most people, body image falls along a continuum. In other words, there are *degrees* to which a person feels negatively or positively about his or her own body—it is usually not just one or the other. Additionally, most people's self-perceptions about body image shift frequently, even on a daily basis. Some, however, may hold extreme, persistently negative views about their bodies, as is often the case with anorexia patients. In severe cases such as these, negative body image may be coupled with *body image distortion.* Body image distortion involves a misperception of body shape and size, and/or a misperception of certain features of the body (e.g., stomach or thighs may inaccurately seem disproportionate to the rest of the body). Perhaps a helpful way of understanding body image distortion is to imagine seeing yourself in a funhouse mirror (see Figure 4). Now imagine perceiving yourself like this on a regular basis; this is perhaps the most fitting description of body image distortion.

Body Image Concerns

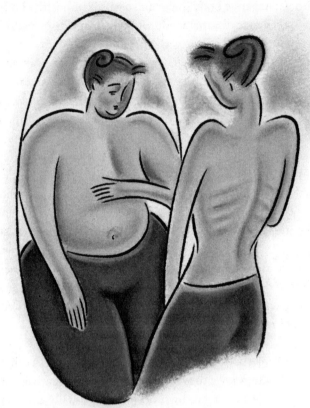

Figure 4   An Illustration of Body Image Distortion
SOURCE: www.gettyimages.com

Sarah shares:

Sometimes people have this idea that patients with anorexia look in a mirror and see something entirely different than what is actually there. The way I see it, if you look at anything under a microscope, it eventually will look big. I scrutinized every single part of my body to the point that even when I was emaciated, all I could see were the imperfections in myself.

44. How do I know if I have a healthy body image?

Keeping in mind that positive and negative body image are on a continuum, you can use the following questionnaire to help guide your thinking about body image acceptance. As you read each statement, respond with one of the following answers: *Always, Frequently, Sometimes,* or *Never.* You may want to write your answers down as you go.*

1) When I look in the mirror, I dislike what I see.
2) The way I treat my body is a result of my frustration with my physical appearance (example: I exercise to "punish" my body because I feel fat or didn't perform well athletically).
3) I think of the worth of myself and my body in terms of appearance (example: I like myself because I look good to-day), not in terms of how it feels and what it does for me (example: I like myself because I am healthy or strong).
4) Even when others tell me I look fine, I think they are lying.
5) When I look in the mirror, I can't help but concentrate on the parts of my body that I dislike or hate.
6) I avoid social situations because of fear, self-consciousness, and anxiety about my body (example: I didn't attend a pool party because of fear of wearing a bathing suit).
7) I do not like being seen in revealing or tight clothing because I am uncomfortable with my body.
8) I think that if I were thinner, I would be happy.
9) I spend a large part of my time thinking about food, weight, calories, and/or appearance.
10) I am afraid of gaining weight or being fat.
11) To me, a good day is one when I feel or look thin, and a bad day is one when I feel or look fat.

If you answered *Always, Frequently,* or *Sometimes* to three or more of these statements, you may be suffering from poor body image. If you answered *Never* to most of the questions, you likely have a healthy, positive body image. Either way, read on to learn about ways to improve your body image.

---

* This questionnaire has been provided by the Multiservice Eating Disorders Association (MEDA) and is used with permission.

Accepting our bodies can be a key toward recovery and good health. After all, you can't love your body too much; it's the only one you've got!

45. What are some of the risk factors for developing body image disturbance?

Many of the risk factors related to body image disturbance are shared risk factors for anorexia. For example, media influence, family and peer influence, depression, anxiety, low self-esteem, poor coping skills, and teasing about weight are shared risk factors (see Questions 22, 24, and 25). Pubertal development may also influence body image, with early developing females and late-developing males reporting more dissatisfaction. Additionally, studies show that pregnancy is a potential risk factor for body image disturbance. According to the *Handbook of Eating Disorders and Obesity,* those at greatest risk for body concerns during the postpartum period are those who retain pregnancy weight and who had body image concerns before their pregnancy. Finally, research indicates that those who engage in comparisons with others regarding weight and body shape are also at greater risk for body image disturbance.

46. What is Body Dysmorphic Disorder?

Body Dysmorphic Disorder (BDD) is perhaps the most severe form of body image disturbance. It is described in the *DSM-IV-TR* as a preoccupation with some imagined defect in physical appearance or an excessive concern with a minor physical irregularity. For example, a person may have severe distress over one or more areas of their body: a facial feature, skin blemish, or body hair; or maybe their head, thighs, stomach, breast, or buttocks. Common complaints associated with BDD involve real or imagined acne, wrinkles, thinning hair, scars, swelling, or facial asymmetry. Also common are concerns with the shape or size of a body part such as the nose, eyes, ears, mouth, jaw, chin, cheeks, or head.

In BDD, the preoccupation with a perceived flaw is excessive and causes significant distress or impairment in functioning. Most people with BDD find their preoccupations difficult to control, to the point that thoughts about their "defect" come to dominate their lives. In order to cope with their distress, many with BDD will continually ask for reassurance from others about their perceived flaw. Some people engage in excessive grooming behaviors and self-scrutiny (e.g., checking themselves frequently with a mirror or magnifying glass) in an attempt to temporarily decrease anxiety about their perceived flaw; however, this generally leads to further preoccupation and distress. Others avoid mirrors altogether out of low self-esteem, shame, embarrassment, or fear of rejection. BDD may lead to social isolation, work problems, and avoidance of social interactions. In extreme cases, individuals may only leave their house at night or become housebound altogether. Some with BDD will attempt to correct their "defect" through cosmetic surgeries; however, these procedures may actually cause the disorder to worsen and lead to an even greater preoccupation with appearance. The distress associated with BDD can lead to hospitalization, suicidal thoughts, and suicide.

BDD affects up to 2% of the U.S. population, affecting both males and females in equal numbers. Symptoms of the disorder usually begin in adolescence or childhood (70% of cases begin before age 18); however, the condition may go undiagnosed for years, perhaps because individuals experiencing symptoms associated with BDD are reluctant to express their concerns with others. Many BDD patients have a co-occurring condition, such as depression, anxiety, or obsessive-compulsive disorder.

As noted in *Eating Disorders and Obesity: A Comprehensive Handbook, Second Edition,* BDD and eating disorders have some obvious similarities, such as a preoccupation with perceived flaws of appearance, a disturbance in body image, and a sense that one's body is unacceptable. However, for patients with BDD, the focus tends to be more on specific body parts than on body shape or weight. According to the *DSM-IV-TR*, a person can receive *both* a diagnosis of BDD and anorexia if warranted, but a person is *not* diagnosed with BDD if their preoccupation and distress is only restricted to "fatness." This person's diagnosis would focus solely on the appropriate eating disorder.

BDD is generally considered a chronic condition with a high rate of relapse. Research on this disorder is in its infancy, although two treatment methods have been identified as being helpful: cognitive-behavioral therapy (see Question 86) and certain psychiatric medications. Both have been shown to decrease the symptoms and distress associated with BDD.

47. How does a healthcare professional assess for and treat body image disturbance?

Assessment can be accomplished through patient interview, combined with the use of various professional assessment materials. In a clinical interview, one's healthcare professional may inquire about a patient's weight history (i.e., current, highest, lowest, longest standing body weight) and subjective satisfaction with weight and body image. The interview may also screen for a history of teasing about appearance and weight, family history of eating disorders, body image dissatisfaction, patient eating disorder behavior, body checking behavior, and other issues salient to body image. Self-report questionnaires are often used to assess body image disturbance and dissatisfaction, such as the one offered in Question 44. Additional self-report questionnaires can be found in *The Body Image Workbook* by Thomas Cash.

In addition, scientific research has yielded a number of useful measures that utilize figure drawings to assess for body image disturbance. These measures involve viewing a series of artist sketches featuring male or female figures. Participants are then asked to respond to questions that pertain to their

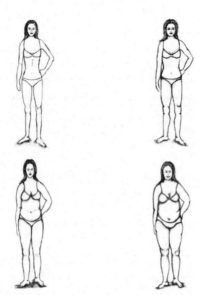

Figure 5   Sample Figures from the Bi-Dimensional Body Evaluation Scale for Women
SOURCE: Ryan, W. J., Sanftner, J. L., and Pierce, P. (2005, June). Validity and reliability of a new visual rating tool for assessing body image in women. Paper presented at the annual meeting of the American College of Sports Medicine, Nashville, Tennessee. Used with permission.

perception of the figures. An example of this type of measure is the *Bidimensional Body Evaluation Scale for Women* (BBESW) (see Figures 5 and 6). The BBESW consists of 32 figures that vary in body fatness and muscularity. Patients are shown the figure array, which is printed on an 8½′ × 11″ sheet of paper, and are asked to respond to the following questions:

1. Which figure do you *think* you look like most of the time?
2. Which figure would you *most like to look like*, in an ideal world?
3. Which figure do you think the social environment (society, friends, TV, magazines, movies, etc.) wants you to look like?
4. Which figure do you think men find most attractive?
5. Which figure do you think women find most attractive?

Body Image Concerns

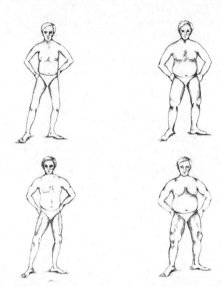

Figure 6   Sample Figures from the Bi-Dimensional Body Evaluation Scale for Men
SOURCES: Ryan, W. J., Sanftner, J. L., and Pierce, P. (2004, June). Validity and reliability of a new visual rating tool for assessing body image in men. Paper presented at the annual meeting of the American College of Sports Medicine, Indianapolis, Indiana. Used with permission.
Ryan, W., Sanftner, J., and Pierce, P. (2002, November). Development of a new visual rating tool for assessing body image in men. Paper presented at the annual meeting of the Mid-Atlantic Regional Chapter of the American College of Sports Medicine, Bushkill, Pennsylvania.
Pierce, P., Ryan, W., and Sanftner, J. L. (2004, March). Anthropometric value associated with self-reported body image using a new visual rating tool. Paper presented at the annual meeting of the American Alliance for Health Physical Education, Recreation, and Dance, New Orleans, Louisiana.

Various therapeutic techniques have shown promise for improving body image perception. Some are experiential in nature. For example, in order to help patients understand the phenomenon of body image distortion, some therapists will ask them to draw an outline of how they think their body looks on a large piece of butcher paper. The therapist will then tape the paper up on a wall and literally trace the outline of their patient's body shape on the paper while he or she stands against it. The patient is then asked to turn around and view the difference between their *perceived* body image, as he or she drew it, and their *actual* body size. Other therapeutic techniques include guided imagery, talk therapy, behavioral interventions, and self-help manuals; each has yielded some measure of success.

A treatment approach increasing in popularity is cognitive-behavioral therapy (CBT). According to psychologist Thomas Cash, CBT treatment of body image issues has been shown to result in increased body satisfaction, decreased investment in appearance, reduced body image distress, and an improvement in the areas of self-esteem, social functioning, and eating behaviors. Cognitive-behavioral therapy includes a psycho-education component that helps patients understand how altering one's thoughts about body image and appearance can lead to decreased body image disturbance and a healthier approach to body shape, appearance, and weight. Cognitive-behavioral therapy utilizes a variety of exercises, including relaxation techniques, journaling, behavior modification, and "homework" exercises aimed at improving body image acceptance and modifying distorted personal beliefs about body image, shape, weight, and appearance.

48. What are some practical ways to improve body image?

There are a number of things a person can do at home to improve body image and reduce body dissatisfaction. However, depending on the person's level of body image disturbance, professional support and treatment may be warranted. This is especially true if eating disorder symptoms are present.

The following is a list of helpful suggestions for building a healthy, positive body image. Although one list cannot automatically tell you how to turn negative thoughts about body image into positive ones, it can be a step toward appreciating, respecting, and valuing yourself and the body that you have been given:*

---

* Special thanks to Dr. Margo Maine and the Multiservice Eating Disorders Association (MEDA) for their contributions to this answer.

— **Recognize** that bodies come in all different shapes and sizes. There is no one "right" body size. Your body is not, and should not be, like anyone else's.

— **Appreciate** all that your body can do. Honor it. Respect it. Fuel it.

— **Focus.** Create a list of all the things your body lets you do. Read it and add to it often. Remember that your body is the instrument of your life, not just an ornament.

— **Socialize.** Don't let your weight or shape keep you from activities that you enjoy.

— **Count** your blessings, not your blemishes.

— **Be** your body's friend and supporter, not its enemy. Care for it.

— **Express gratitude.** Every morning when you wake up, thank your body for resting and rejuvenating itself so you can enjoy the day. Every evening when you go to bed, tell your body how much you appreciate what it has allowed you to do throughout the day.

— **Keep** a list of positive things about yourself—without mentioning your appearance. Add to it, and read it often. Choose to find beauty in the world and in yourself.

— **Consider** getting rid of the scale. It's what's inside that counts.

— **Remember** that your size, shape, and weight do not determine your worth as a person. You are not just your body.

— **Become** a critical viewer of the media. Begin to question whether the sculpted images of men and waiflike images of women are realistic. Pay attention to images, slogans, or attitudes that make you feel bad about yourself or your body. Protest these messages: Write a letter to the advertiser or talk back to the image or message.

— **Think** about all of the things you could accomplish for others with the time and energy you spend worrying about your body and appearance. Try one! Reaching out to help another person can be a great way to make a positive change in our world and to feel better about yourself!

— **Surround** yourself with positive people who care about your well-being. Find friends who are not overly concerned with body weight and appearance.

— **Talk.** When you are feeling badly, talk about it!

49. What can I do to enhance my child's body image?

One important step toward enhancing your child's body image is to examine your feelings and attitudes about *your own* body image. How did you feel about your body growing up? Do you compare your body to others'? Do you diet frequently? Do you make disparaging comments about your own weight or appearance? Do you exercise only for the purpose of losing weight or burning off calories that you ate in "excess"? If so, your son or daughter will take notice. While you may not intend to "pass down" negative feelings about body image, weight, and appearance, your children will look to you as a model for what it is like to relate to one's own body.

Secondly, withhold negative comments about appearance or weight, both your own *and* your child's. If you are self-conscious about your own weight and appearance, whatever the reason, your child is more likely to be as well. Help your child gain a sense of self-esteem and self-worth that is not based primarily on appearance, weight, or body shape. Examining your own attitudes about these issues will go a long way toward achieving that goal.

Next, be affirming in your comments about your child's strengths. Your child may not always seem responsive to your gestures of support, but they do not go unnoticed. Encourage broad varieties of activities, strengths, and achievements in order to place importance on what your children *do* and who your children *are*, rather than on their appearance. Help your children learn assertive communication, and teach them to

Your children will look to you as a model for what it is like to relate to one's own body.

Body Image Concerns

stand up for their rights as individuals—especially their right to be treated with dignity and seen as *whole, complete people,* valued for things that go beyond their appearance, such as their contributions to their world and community.

Finally, balance is a key. Be sure to have a balanced approach to exercise and nutrition in the home. Maintain an informed view of the media and the many societal pressures to be thin. Discuss these things with your children, and encourage open, honest dialogue about the pressures regarding weight and appearance they may be facing in their social circles, school environments, or athletic groups. Help your children understand the natural changes to body shape and appearance that occur during puberty, and help them to appreciate the ways in which their bodies are changing and growing. Learn about the signs and symptoms to watch out for with regard to eating disordered behavior, but also celebrate the positive at the same time! Support their efforts to develop positive regard for themselves, *and* their bodies!

PART SEVEN

Support for Loved Ones

I know caring for my child will be a challenge, but I'm not sure what to expect. What type of difficulties might I face?

I feel ashamed to tell any of my friends about my child's eating disorder. I'm not sure I would know what to say even if I tried. What should I do?

Our family therapist said my child needs to gain weight, but should I be weighing her at home to track her progress?

More . . .

50. My daughter was recently diagnosed with anorexia, and, needless to say, I am overwhelmed. My life feels like it has been turned upside down. I am scared and tired, but at the same time, I desperately want to be there for her. How can I get through this?

Getting help for your child is critically important because you cannot do this alone. She will need the help of caring professionals, as we have discussed earlier. However, it is perhaps equally important for you to receive help and support as well. Caring for a person with anorexia can be a very challenging task, and regardless of the severity of the disorder, the diagnosis of anorexia in a loved one brings questions, fears, and concerns that should not be overlooked. It is important to reduce any feeling of isolation that you may be experiencing. Thus, having a place to discuss your concerns, process your feelings, and find support for yourself can be a valuable means of assistance.

It is important to reduce any feeling of isolation that you may be experiencing.

Many parents find it helpful to talk with other parents of anorexia patients. Families learn how to lean on each other for support, listen to each other's challenges, and glean helpful advice for handling the family changes that come with a loved one's eating disorder. Resources such as the Parents, Family and Friends Network (PFN) at the National Eating Disorders Association and the Family and Friends Support Finder at *www.something-fishy.org* provide means for building connections between parents of anorexia patients. Parental support groups are available, both those led by professional therapists and those led by other concerned parents. The National Association of Anorexia Nervosa and Associated Disorders (ANAD) offers free support groups in many parts of the United States, some of which are open to family members. If there are no local support groups in your area, consider starting one yourself. Many of the organizations listed in the Resources section of this book may be able to help you begin a group and provide resources for doing so.

In addition, loved ones often find that personal and/or family therapy is a helpful tool and source of support. A trained therapist can help family members gain answers to questions, discuss personal feelings, learn to accept personal limitations, and work through interpersonal conflict.

Lastly, consider some of the other resources that can help families arm themselves with education about anorexia. *Eating Disorders Today* (published by Gürze Books) is a quarterly newsletter geared toward helping recovering individuals *and* their loved ones. Blogs, chat rooms, and online support groups lead the way in new technologies as sources of family support. Toll-free help lines are available as well (see the Resources section for more information).

51. I know caring for my child will be a challenge, but I'm not sure what to expect. What type of difficulties might I face?

While each anorexia patient faces his or her own unique challenges, timeline for recovery, and illness severity, the burden on family members can be great regardless of these factors. As a result, caregivers often report high levels of unmet needs of their own. According to *Eating Disorders Review*, studies show that a family's burden while caring for a loved one with anorexia may be comparable to caring for someone with other forms of persistent mental illness. Caregivers may face additional challenges with co-occurring conditions in loved ones, such as depression, anxiety, substance abuse, or self-injury. All of these reasons reinforce the need for loved ones to have sufficient support for themselves.

Family members commonly report having to deal with issues such as disruption of family mealtimes, increased emotional conflict, defiance on the part of a child anorexia patient, and increased social isolation. Some parents report strain on their marriage, strain in their relationships with their other children, and complicated sibling relationships as the result of anorexia in the family. Simple acts such as shopping for groceries can become increasingly complicated as parents are unsure of how to handle a child's unusual demands and restrictions with regard to food in the home. Family members may face their own illnesses, mental health needs, marital strife, divorce adjustment, or work problems that warrant attention. Caring for a person with anorexia can be a complicated task; however, the right resources and a strong treatment team will enable you to face any challenges ahead with increased confidence.

Sarah shares:

When I was sick, everyone around me felt so out of control and frustrated with me, like I wasn't listening to anything they had to say. Little did they know, I felt almost as powerless as they did. I didn't know what else to do except listen to my eating disorder. But it's hard to explain that to your mom when she makes your favorite meal and you refuse to eat it, or to your friends when you repeatedly back out of plans because you know it will involve food at some point.

I yelled, cursed, and threw things at my mother—things I never would have done had I been in my right mind. These behaviors only came out at my worst times, and my mom had to learn to see through my destructive actions and realize that my eating disorder was controlling me; it simply wasn't me acting so badly.

52. What do you hear most often from the parents of anorexia patients regarding their experiences? What can I learn from other parents who are facing the same struggles?

In speaking with parents of anorexia patients over the years, I have watched many families overcome great struggles and come through difficulties to be even stronger than when they began their journey of caring for a loved one in recovery. I have seen family members learn from each other and offer support to each other in remarkable ways. Wise counsel can be taken from their experiences and through the knowledge they gained amidst very trying circumstances. Some of their "pearls of wisdom" I gladly share with you now:

- "I learned not to blame myself. Anorexia is not my fault."
- "Anorexia is an illness. When I finally 'got' that, it helped me to stop blaming my child, my husband, and the world for her condition. It helped me to better support her recovery."
- "Learning to listen, *really listen,* to my son was difficult to do because I just wanted him to stop the eating disorder. Letting him talk about his feelings turned out to be the best thing I could do for him, and it brought healing to our family."
- "Setting limits was hard at first because I felt so guilty doing it. But my daughter was running our household with all of her food restrictions, and I needed to set limits in a loving way so we could function well as a family."
- "I learned that taking care of my needs while my child was sick was important too. It was really helpful to have support from other people."
- "I finally realized that I couldn't do it all. I needed help, and when I got the courage to ask for it, it started to make a difference."
- "Don't take their angry words at you personally" (spoken by a sister of an anorexia patient).
- "I stopped being ashamed—of myself as a mother, or of my daughter's illness. It sounds obvious, but it took some work on my part."
- "Have family time together that doesn't focus on food" (spoken by a teen patient in recovery).
- "I am a good mother, and I love my child. Anorexia did not change that—but it did help to remind myself sometimes."

Doris Smeltzer, an educator for nearly 20 years, was thrust into the world of eating disorders through Andrea, her 19-year-old daughter, who died from an eating disorder in 1999. Since her daughter's death, Doris cofounded, with her husband Tom, the non-profit eating disorders prevention foundation Andrea's Voice. Doris also authors a blog entitled "Advice for Parents" at *www.eatingdisordersblogs.com*. In it, she lists some of the things she would have liked, as a parent, to have received from a treatment team regarding her daughter's eating disorder. With Doris' permission, I have included some of her "wishes" here so that readers might learn from her experience. Doris writes:

It would have been helpful to me if members of a treatment team had:

1. told me that the eating disorder did not intend to go away quietly and that it could take my child with it.
2. explained to me why my child could not think rationally by educating me about the effects of starvation, bingeing, and purging on the brain and body.
3. helped me understand that my child could not begin the arduous task of giving up her eating disorder until she was capable of rational thought.
4. explored characteristics in me that mirrored my child's. This would have helped me examine and begin to change my own perfectionism, all or nothing thinking, and/or tendency to put the care of others before my own self-care, which would have made me better able to help my child do the same.
5. modeled and discussed ways that we, as a mother and a father, could have celebrated our own body types.

6. encouraged me to grieve the family of times past and the past experience of, and relationship with, my child. This may have allowed me to focus on the *now* and helped me see how as a family we could work together to create a future that included more helpful ways of being in a relationship.

7. validated for me that pain is a fact of life but that I did not have to suffer. This would have helped me to develop strategies or to find resources that supported me in ways that might have alleviated or reduced my suffering.

In addition, and in hindsight, Doris adds to her "wish list" the following:

- I wish I had truly understood how emotionally and psychologically addictive were her behaviors.
- I wish I had known that a person can look and feel fantastic and be close to death.
- I wish I had recognized that Andrea being cold all the time was a sign of hypothermia.
- I wish I had been told that the long, feathery eyelashes I one day noticed in the last weeks of her life were a warning sign. Lanugo, the baby-fine hair that often covers the bodies of those who are starving, can manifest itself in the eyelashes. Andrea did not look starved.
- I wish I had not accepted our culture's "normalization" of diets. I thought Andrea's preoccupation with weight and body size were normal "rites of passage" that would recede with time, as mine had. Andrea was not me.
- I wish with all my heart I had been more of a parent and less of a friend in the final months

of Andrea's life. As her friend, I lost my objectivity. My empathy for her led, at times, to a subtle and inadvertent support of her disease. How I wish I could change that reality!

I would like to thank Doris and Tom for their generosity in sharing this information and for the hope they provide to families who are caring for a loved one in recovery. You can learn more about Doris's journey of self-discovery in the book *Andrea's Voice: Silenced by Bulimia.*

53. I feel ashamed to tell any of my friends about my child's eating disorder. I'm not sure I would know what to say even if I tried. What should I do?

Sharing with others that your child has an eating disorder can feel like revealing an intimate secret. Some families express shame in telling others because of the unfortunate stigma associated with the illness. Parents may feel afraid they will be blamed for their child's illness. Loved ones may feel offended by comments made in response to their disclosure. However, telling others can actually be an antidote to stigma and blame, especially when one is able to correct misconceptions about anorexia. While there are no guarantees that your friends will completely understand what you are going through, many of them will likely want to help when given the opportunity.

Telling others can actually be an antidote to stigma and blame.

You may want to speak with your child before sharing with others so that there can be a consensus as to how much information is shared. Your child may need reassurance that you will only share with those you trust. Explain what information will be shared, with whom, along with your purpose for sharing. Let your child know that you feel it will be helpful to the family to have outside support. Be prepared for questions from others, but don't fear them. If questions get too personal, or if you receive any unwanted advice, do not hesitate to set appropriate boundaries. You always have the option of simply saying, "Thank you for your concern. My child is getting the help she needs. I appreciate your support."

54. Lately it feels like our lives revolve around our son's anorexia. Our household rules have nearly dissolved to the point of confusion and chaos. We're unsure how much we should adhere to his demands with regard to mealtimes and the type of food we serve. Can you give us some help that might take us in the right direction?

Your request is quite common. Many families are unsure how to navigate the many rules, food restrictions, and mealtime rituals that beset the home of an anorexia patient. Frequently, parents and siblings try to arrange the kitchen, grocery shopping lists, and mealtime habits around the behaviors of a person with an eating disorder in an attempt to "keep the peace" and avoid arguments. Making these accommodations may also be a way to try to reduce patient distress or relieve feelings of blame or guilt on the part of healthy family members. However, although these adjustments may seem helpful in the short term, they may actually increase household tensions, sibling resentment, and caregiver burden over time.

According to *Surviving an Eating Disorder: Strategies for Family and Friends,* it is important that as parents, you *do set household rules and expectations* in order to convey that your child's eating disorder will not take over your family's life. For example, although it may be tempting, do not purchase or avoid purchasing certain foods solely to accommodate a patient's demands. Your child is not the only one to eat in your home, and each person's nutritional needs must be met. You may hear many demands from your child with regard to what food is purchased for the home, how food is prepared, how food is stored, how dishes and utensils are cleaned, who does the cooking, whether or not conversation should take place at the dinner table, how much money is spent on food, and so on. If a family begins to pattern their behaviors around eating disordered "rules" such as these, it can lead to habits that become difficult to change. Contrary to how it may seem, allowing such demands will not reduce your child's food anxiety but will likely lead to increased food anxiety and, in turn, additional rules and restrictions.

You may find it helpful to work with your child's treatment team in deciding what limits will work best in your unique situation, limits that will respect the needs of *every* family member and convey love, care, and concern for your child's recovery—not enable eating disordered behaviors. Finding a balance can indeed be a challenge, but there are some general things to keep in mind when setting household rules:

- Discuss your reasoning openly with your child. He or she may not understand or even be willing to accept your decisions, but being open with your child will convey a sense of love and respect.
- Whenever possible, involve all family members working together. Maintaining boundaries is a team effort, and families need support from one another to do so.
- Be consistent. It may be tempting to allow breaking of the rules, especially when you are tired or feeling frustrated. However, this can perpetuate unhealthy patterns and reward misbehavior.
- Be flexible and open to negotiations around rules. For example, if your child with anorexia does not want to do certain household tasks that involve food, consider allowing a replacement chore for them that causes less discomfort.
- Remain calm. Do not let the family table become a battleground. Set loving limits and consequences for acting out, in the same way you would with your other children. This will also help to reduce sibling confusion and resentment.

- Healthy siblings should not "take over" chores for an ill child, as this can lead to resentment and additional conflict. In addition, studies show that healthy siblings can experience feelings of loss, anxiety, and depression if too little attention is given to them when a sibling is ill, so take pleasure in spending time with all of your children and reassuring them of your love and attention.
- Know your limitations. You cannot "argue" your child out of an eating disorder. Remember that if your child is in a state of semi-starvation, he or she may not be able to respond to reason.
- Allow for acceptable independence. Do not force your child to eat or bribe them into eating.
- Maintain clear boundaries. If your child offends another family member or engages in behavior that disregards another person's rights or feelings, allow for consequences and correction as you would for your other children.
- If you find that you are experiencing frequent feelings of guilt, or in contrast, feelings of resentment toward your child, talk with a therapist or other supportive professional.

55. My wife has become more irritable and withdrawn since she became ill with anorexia, and I have difficulty communicating with her. Her eating disorder symptoms seem to compound this problem so that when we do talk, it's often about her weight concerns. How do I talk comfortably with her?

Communication is an important part of any marriage or familial relationship, and many parents, siblings, children, and friends would echo your uncertainty of how to communicate effectively with an anorexia patient. Unfortunately, as you have observed, anorexia can limit a person's ability to engage in meaningful exchanges, both because of the preoccupation with food and weight and because of the physiological effects of starvation and the resulting cognitive and affective changes. Marital therapy can be quite helpful and is highly recommended, if your spouse is willing to attend. If that is not feasible, I can suggest some strategies for encouraging effective communication in marital and other familial relationships:

- Openly express your love and affection for your spouse or loved one.
- Listen to her feelings without judgment. Try to reflect what you hear her saying to you (e.g., "I hear you saying that you feel scared" or "I am hearing you say that you feel you must be perfect").
- Show compassion and empathy for her feelings. You can do this without agreeing with the beliefs your loved one holds about food and weight.
- Do not get drawn in to questions about weight and conversations about food. Instead, attempt to gently guide the conversation to other topics (entertainment, a planned activity, or another subject of interest to your loved one). Sharing in non-food related activities can be a source of pleasure for both of you and may allow for a wider range of conversation as well.
- Do not try to read your loved one's mind. If you want to know what he or she is feeling or thinking, ask directly.
- If an argument ensues, take a break from the conversation and come back to it when you are both calmer. Do not simply insist that your viewpoint is correct; instead attempt to understand all points of view, even though you may not agree.
- Disagreements are okay. It can be healthy for couples to have and express their varying opinions. Insist on mutual respect at all times.
- Avoid blaming the other person or making accusatory statements such as "If you would just eat, we wouldn't have any problems." Do not try to induce guilt. Do not try to argue or lecture your loved one into changing his

or her behavior. Do not threaten the withdrawal of your love or affection.

- Do not give advice, unless requested.
- Avoid exaggerations such as "you *always*" or "you *never.*"
- Be willing to acknowledge your own mistakes in an argument, and do not hesitate to apologize for them.
- Try using "feeling language" or "I" statements, which are ways of expressing how *you* feel about a situation without placing blame on another. For example, the statements "*you* are slipping again" or "*you* are in danger of purging" can make your spouse feel defensive or hostile. "I" statements can help you communicate your *own* feelings and experiences, not another's (e.g., "*I* am worried about what I have been witnessing lately" or "*I* get scared when you say you think you are fat"). The key is to discuss your own feelings without trying to assume what the other person is feeling. As a basic guideline for "I" statements, you can try following this three-part format:

1. I feel _____ (name your feeling)
2. When _____ (provide nonjudgmental description of behavior)
3. Because _____ (give the effect the behavior has on you or on others).

Example: *I feel* upset *when* you withdraw to the other room at dinner time *because* the kids and I don't get to have your company.

56. What about eating out? My family used to do this regularly, but now my son doesn't want to go with us because of his eating disorder. Should I insist he go?

The experience of eating out in a restaurant can indeed be a very positive one, and many people enjoy doing so frequently. Just look at the popularity of eating out as a social experience—on dates, for special occasions, and as family outings. However, for the person with anorexia, social eating can be

For the person with anorexia, social eating can be fraught with intense feelings of fear, anxiety, and shame.

fraught with intense feelings of fear, anxiety, and shame. Asking your son about his specific concerns may give way to a resolution. For example, you may ask him if there are any restaurants in which he would feel "safe" and comfortable. Let him choose one accordingly. It may be hard to understand his reasoning, but try asking your son what his feelings are on the matter and listening to his response—it could open up lines of communication in a new way.

Food exchange system

A dietary approach or special meal plan in which foods are categorized by food group (e.g., starches, vegetables) and serving size.

If he is using a **food exchange system**, his dietitian may be able to provide helpful advice for applying this information to social eating situations. If a compromise cannot be reached, then for now, it may be best to respect his wishes on the matter. Try not to take his decision personally; instead remember that it is a symptom of his anorexia and will likely change as he takes strides in recovery. As your son progresses in treatment, he will probably once again become comfortable with eating in social situations.

57. I'm concerned about my college roommate. I really think she has an eating disorder, but I'm scared to approach her. What should I do?

First, you may wish to refer to Question 12 to determine if your concern is warranted. If so, there are a few tips that may help. As a way of remembering a few key pieces of information, I created the acronym *ALIVE* for using a caring approach in speaking with a loved one about anorexia:

*A*sk to speak to your loved one in private.
*L*et your loved one know what makes you feel concerned (e.g., discuss specific times when you observed symptoms or behaviors that led to your concern).
*I*nvite your loved one to examine helpful resources about eating disorders and to speak with a caring professional who is knowledgeable about eating disorders. It can be helpful to come prepared with names of Web sites, books, or local treatment professionals (see the Resources section).

*V*oice your concerns without engaging in a power struggle, assigning blame, or offering simple solutions (e.g., "If you would just eat, everything would be fine"). *E*xpress your desire to support your loved one. Remind them of your love and of your concern for their well-being.

Keep in mind that your goal for sharing is to encourage your roommate to get help. Toward that end, there are a few more things to consider. First, try not to argue with her if she refuses to get help. Instead, express how it makes you feel to see her engaging in behaviors that may be harmful to her health. Using "I" statements can be helpful here (see Question 55). If it appears the conversation may turn into an intense argument, simply suggest that you talk about the matter again at another time. Realistically, you do need to prepare yourself for the possibility that your roommate may react in denial or become angry at your suggestion to get help. Instead of trying to push for change, reinforce that you are there for her should she ever wish to talk about it again, then consider backing away from the issue temporarily.

Second, give your roommate the opportunity to respond to your concerns. Perhaps she will welcome the display of care and concern you show. You can ask if there is anything you can do to be helpful; however, know your limitations. Do not attempt to give professional advice or take on a role beyond that which would be appropriate to your relationship. Be sure to direct your roommate to speak with a school nurse, coach, teacher, or parent. Third, if the situation calls for an emergency response, do not hesitate. If you are aware of the potential for a suicide attempt or physical harm due to the effects of starvation, assist your roommate in getting appropriate help at a hospital or other urgent care facility.

Wishing to avoid offense, wanting to not appear intrusive, and fearing angry responses are frequent reasons why people hesitate to share concerns with others. However, while you are under no obligation to share your concerns, your helpful action may steer your roommate toward getting help.

The knowledge that someone is willing to offer helpful resources and come alongside as a caring source of support can be a powerful impetus toward getting help. If you feel you can no longer keep your concerns to yourself, I hope the information presented here will help you prepare to speak with your roommate.

Sarah shares:

When approaching a friend who you think might be in trouble, expect the worst. Even when I sincerely wanted help, I responded to people who reached out to me by brushing off their concern or getting mad at them for "falsely" accusing me of being sick.

No matter how stubborn and mean your friend is, don't *give up on them. Understand that deep down, they don't want to push you away and refuse your help. Let them know you're not going anywhere, and when they get angry with you, know that it is their eating disorder talking, not them.*

58. Our family therapist said my child needs to gain weight, but should I be weighing her at home to track her progress?

While weight checks are necessary to track a patient's progress toward weight restoration, it is often best if they are conducted by the treatment team, rather than at home. In fact, you may consider getting rid of the at-home scale for the time being. Frequent weighing can be a source of stress and anxiety for an anorexia patient and can actually serve to increase food- and weight-related obsessions. Patients have been known to hide a scale and weigh themselves often, sometimes hourly—a habit that is clearly unproductive for recovery. If your child's treatment team instructs you to conduct weight checks at home (once per week, at most), try having your child step onto the scale backward so that he or she is unable to read the number on the scale; that way you will be able to see how your child is progressing toward targeted treatment goals without sharing specifics.

59. Our daughter has been in recovery for 2 years now and is doing well. She wants to go away to college in the fall, but we're not sure it is a good idea yet. What should we consider when making this decision?

You may wish to garner the assistance of your child's treatment team for this important decision. Each member of the team will be able to offer valuable input as to your child's level of readiness, dietary concerns, warning signs to consider, and potential emotional triggers to be aware of when your child is away from home. Eating disorders are more prevalent on college campuses than in the general population. In addition, the stress of leaving home and living in an unfamiliar environment, and the challenges of **individuation** are factors that can serve as triggers for an increase in eating disorder symptoms. Another important consideration is whether your child has developed the sufficient coping skills necessary for self-care. Usually, it is best for a person in recovery to wait to go to college until he or she has returned to a healthy weight, has demonstrated normal eating patterns, has a balanced approach to exercise and nutrition, and has acquired sufficient skills for managing daily stress. You may wish to ensure that your child does not take on too many courses or social commitments too soon and/or arrange a "Plan B" alternative schedule should the experience become overwhelming. You may also wish to provide reassurance that returning home is an option if your child decides he or she is not yet ready to live away at college.

Ideally, you should connect your child to the college student health center or a local treatment professional *before* he or she leaves for school. This is a much better alternative than waiting until a potential crisis arises before connecting to local resources. Additionally, telephone contact can be maintained between your child and his or her home-based treatment team while a relationship with local professionals is being established. Prior to leaving home, you may wish to role-play

Individuation

The developmental process of forming one's individual personality.

some scenarios with your child; for example, you may work through what to do if his or her roommate has an eating disorder, or what to do if he or she experiences some minor setbacks in progress. Finally, maintain open communication between you and your child while he or she is away. Keep in mind, however, that with certain exceptions, if your child is over the age of 18, unless he or she makes allowances for you to communicate with his or her local treatment team, the information shared between the team and your child will remain confidential (see Question 91).

60. What are some practical suggestions for families of loved ones dealing with anorexia nervosa?

Many families find it helpful to have a list of "do's" and "don'ts." I have included one here to which you can refer as needed.

Things *to do* when a loved one has anorexia or another eating disorder:

- Understand all you can about this complex illness.
- Obtain adequate self-support to ensure you have the coping skills needed to care for your loved one. Know your own limitations.
- Expand your list of resources for information and support (see the Resources section of this book for a helpful list).
- Seek appropriate treatment.
- Listen to and heed any recommendations from health-care professionals.
- Maintain contact and open lines of communication with *all* members of the family.
- Encourage positive self-esteem (not based on physical appearance) in your loved one. Support their unique personality, talents, and abilities.
- Sincerely praise any progress in recovery, but *avoid* basing comments on appearance or weight.

- Relate to your loved one as a *person*, rather than relating to their anorexia. Understand that the two are separate.
- Know that recovery can be a long, hard process and can take a significant amount of time and resources.
- Realize there are no quick and easy solutions to an eating disorder.
- Understand there may be times when your help may be rejected or when you cannot bring about change. Remember that your loved one must choose to put in the effort and do the work associated with recovery. You cannot force a person to recover. You can, however, be a consistent source of love and support.
- Maintain clear relationship boundaries.
- Allow your loved one privacy. Resist the temptation to "spy" on his or her eating disorder behavior.
- Strengthen family relationships. It is okay to have enjoyable, fun times as a family, and it may indeed prove quite helpful to do so.
- Maintain an active, supportive social life for yourself. This can help reduce stress levels and offers a great way to "take a break" from the demands of caring for a loved one. It will also help you avoid drifting into isolation and exhaustion. Also allow and encourage supportive friendships in the life of your loved one.
- Set a healthy example. Have a positive, balanced approach to food. Enjoy and respect your own body. Exercise in moderation.
- If your loved one is at an immediate risk of harm, seek emergency intervention.

Things *not to do* when a loved one has anorexia or another eating disorder:

- Do not threaten your loved one if he or she refuses help.
- Do not engage in a power struggle to make your loved one receive help.
- Do not attempt to control the progress of a loved one's recovery.

Support for Loved Ones

- Do not assign blame. Do not criticize or judge your loved one for his or her illness.
- Do not act as "food police."
- Do not make comments about weight or appearance— even your own.
- Do not try to diagnose or treat an eating disorder on your own, apart from the appropriate involvement of a healthcare professional.
- Do not ignore medical risk or complications.
- Do not keep your loved one from socially appropriate activities because of his or her eating disorder. This can lead to further isolation.
- Do not feel obligated to respond directly to weight-related questions such as, "Am I fat?" Instead, remind your love one of your unconditional support and reinforce his or her inner attributes and positive qualities. If you are unsure how to respond to a question, write it down and discuss it with the treatment team.
- Do not deny or ignore your own need for support. Do not ignore other family members' needs for interaction and support. Do not allow a loved one's anorexia to be a distraction or excuse for not attending to your own needs.

Sarah shares:

The best thing I could have hoped for was a positive role model, who for me, came in the form of my mother. Knowing that someone could eat in a healthy way and not lose control of themselves was a great comfort to me when I couldn't do these things for myself.

Even at the worst times, I wanted people to understand that the old, healthy Sarah was still deep down inside me and that I didn't like being the way I was (even if my behavior suggested otherwise). I will always appreciate those people who talked to me like I was still a person, and spoke of my anorexia as a temporary illness that would pass even when it seemed like I would never get better.

PART EIGHT

Weight Restoration, Nutrition, and Healthy Eating

What is nutrition counseling?

What types of foods are included in a healthy, balanced approach to nutrition?

How is weight restoration achieved, and why is it important?

More . . .

61. What is nutrition counseling?

The purpose of **nutrition counseling** includes helping patients enhance their understanding of healthy eating, learn a balanced approach to food, make and maintain dietary changes, and increase motivation to acquire and maintain a healthy weight. Nutrition counseling can also help patients examine underlying beliefs about food, correct any misconceptions or "diet myths," provide an understanding of necessary nutrients for healthy living, assess nutritional imbalances or deficits, and help reestablish a connection to physical hunger and satiety cues that may be significantly impaired by their eating disorder. Knowledgeable nutrition experts (**registered dietitians**, for example) are included in a patient's treatment team to help facilitate these goals. While studies show that nutrition counseling in *isolation* is not an effective treatment for anorexia, and is therefore not recommended, it is highly recommended in *conjunction* with medical and psychological treatment, both for short-term weight recovery as well as to prevent long-term relapse.

Registered dietitian

A qualified, trained, and credentialed expert in food and nutrition.

62. It has been so long that I need to be reminded—what does "healthy eating" look like?

Healthy eating is flexible eating. Healthy eating allows for a wide variety of foods, both for nutritional value as well as for the emotional value of having a balanced, *non-restrictive* approach to eating. Healthy eating yields physical benefits (e.g., clear thinking, mood stability, physical strength, and endurance), and it also allows for the experience of *pleasure* when eating—something that is usually absent for a person with anorexia.

Healthy eating is flexible eating.

According to psychotherapist Karen Koenig, author of *The Rules for Normal Eating*, there is *no one right way* to be a "normal eater." For example, healthy eating may consist of three large meals, or many small ones throughout the day. Koenig adds that "normal" eating means focusing on the food in front of you, rather than worrying about what you ate yesterday or planning what you will eat tomorrow. Healthy eating means not caring what people around you are eating or comparing your portion sizes to theirs. It *excludes* feelings of guilt, shame, or embarrassment, and it does not judge one's *deservingness* when it comes to food and eating. Registered dietitian Ellyn Satter, author of *Secrets of Feeding a Healthy Family: Orchestrating and Enjoying the Family Meal*, sees normal eating as comprised of the following:

- Being able to eat when you are hungry and continue until you are satisfied
- Being able to choose food you like, eat it, and truly get enough of it, not just stop eating because you think you should
- Being able to give some thought to your food selection so you get nutritious food, but not being so wary and restrictive that you miss out on enjoyable food
- Giving yourself permission to eat sometimes because you are happy, sad, or bored, or just because it feels good

In short, healthy eating is not just about what kinds of food you may eat, how often you eat, or how much food you consume; it is also about a healthy *attitude* toward eating—being comfortable with food and being able to eat without fear, judgment, or shame.

Sarah shares:

A huge part of my treatment was learning to eat like a kindergartener—to eat what I wanted when I was hungry—and to stop when my stomach was full (not when my mind told me I should be). I needed a lot of help to relearn which foods I actually liked and which foods I had convinced myself I hated because of their undesirable nutrition facts. After a while, I learned what a healthy portion was and could leave food on my plate if I wanted or go back for seconds if I was still hungry.

63. What types of foods are included in a healthy, balanced approach to nutrition?

Nutrition experts advise including six basic types of nutrients as the building blocks of a healthy diet: carbohydrates, protein, fats, vitamins, minerals, and water. Each of these nutrients provides an important array of benefits to one's health and well-being (a summary of these benefits can be found in Table 3). Your dietitian can assist you in developing a plan that incorporates adequate amounts of key nutrients, energy (calories), and an appropriate proportion of foods for optimal health.

In addition, the U.S. Department of Agriculture (USDA) issued a new set of recommended dietary guidelines in 2005. These guidelines describe a healthy diet as one that: (1) includes a variety of fruits, vegetables, whole grains, and low-fat milk and milk products; (2) is low in saturated fats, **trans fats**, cholesterol, salt (sodium), and added sugars; (3) offers a regular intake of fluids; and (4) includes lean meats, poultry, fish, beans, eggs, and nuts. The intent of the USDA guidelines is to provide science-based advice that promotes good health and to reduce risk for major chronic diseases through diet and physical activity.

Another helpful tool for good nutrition is the Food Pyramid (see Figure 7). Recently, the USDA and the U.S. Department of Health and Human Services developed a new, interactive food pyramid that symbolizes a personalized approach to healthy eating and physical activity. The interactive Web site *www.MyPyramid.gov* allows you to personalize this food pyramid based on your age, gender, and amount of daily physical activity.

Trans fats

Fats that have been treated with hydrogen. Used in many processed foods in order to increase shelf life and flavor stability.

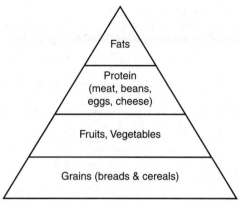

Figure 7   Food Pyramid

64. When my daughter was hospitalized with anorexia, her doctor cautioned us about "refeeding syndrome edema." What is this condition?

Certain serious complications can occur in significantly underweight patients during the course of regaining weight (also called refeeding). These complications result from feeding a severely malnourished patient too much food, too soon. Thus, instead of rapid refeeding, a physician will start a recovering person on small amounts of food and progressively increase the amount of calories consumed. This is true for both oral and **enteral** refeeding.

In refeeding syndrome edema, certain electrolyte disturbances can occur, causing a significant increase in fluid in the blood vessels. As a result, a patient's hands, feet, and ankles may swell. If not properly managed, fluid can build up in the lungs. Abdominal pain, kidney and liver damage, heart failure, and even death can result from refeeding edema and other refeeding complications. The risk of these complications can be minimized or avoided with properly monitored refeeding. Therefore, it is very important that a physician supervise weight restoration in a severely undernourished patient.

Enteral

A method of substance delivery where nutrients are given directly into the gastrointestinal tract.

Weight Restoration, Nutrition, and Healthy Eating

Table 3   Benefits of Key Nutrients

Key Nutrient for Optimal Health	Benefits
Carbohydrates (suggested 45–55% of daily food intake)	• Important part of a balanced diet and the body's preferred source of energy and fuel • Simple carbohydrates (fruits, sugars, honey) are an instant source of energy • Complex carbohydrates (grains, beans, vegetables) are a valuable source of fiber
Protein (suggested 20–30% of daily food intake)	• Assists with tissue repair and maintenance • Supports organ, muscle, and immune functioning • Provides essential amino acids
Fats (suggested 20–30% of daily food intake)	• Are a secondary energy source • Provide essential fatty acids necessary for healthy tissue functioning • Help to regulate body temperature • Protect brain and other organ functioning • Necessary for reproductive health • Aid in satiety
Water (6–8 glasses recommended daily)	• Transports nutrients to cells • Lubricates joints • Aids in digestion
Vitamins	• Assist body with energy utilization
Minerals (e.g., calcium, iron, potassium)	• Aid in bone growth and support • Assist organ functioning • Prevent fatigue • Assist with wound healing • Balance key fluids and electrolytes

A nutrition therapist or dietitian may also assist with refeeding that takes place in a medically supervised environment.

65. How is weight restoration achieved, and why is it important?

Remember that many of the medical, emotional, and social consequences of anorexia nervosa are a result of malnutrition (see Questions 9 and 13). Proper physical and emotional health cannot be attained if a person remains undernourished. Additionally, maintaining a healthy weight is associated with a better treatment outcome and reduces the likelihood of returning to intensive treatment. For these reasons, returning to a healthy weight is an important aspect of recovery.

The approach to weight restoration by a treatment team will depend in part on the severity of a person's illness, medical history, eating disorder symptoms (frequency and severity of restricting food, binging/purging), and nutritional needs. Recommendations and goals regarding weight gain are determined in collaboration with the patient whenever possible. Both for medical reasons and to reduce any anxiety associated with weight gain, weight restoration proceeds incrementally and at a slow pace (generally within the range of 1–4 pounds per week, depending on medical need). Progress can be monitored by the patient, the patient's family, and/or members of the treatment team. Once a healthy weight range is achieved, the focus then shifts to weight maintenance.

Nutritional counseling can help patients learn both *what* to eat as well as *when* to eat in the process of weight restoration. Many people with anorexia report eating at irregular intervals, thus refeeding plans often suggest eating at regularly scheduled times to correct unhealthy patterns. Other aspects of **meal plans** maximize nutrients and health benefits and provide structure and safety while attempting to take into account patient preferences. Depending on the level of care necessary, meal plans may be "structured" (stipulating what to eat, how much to eat, and when to eat), "semi-structured" (offering choices from a list of food groups or food options), or "unstructured" (providing a set caloric or weight-gain goal, but no designed food plan). Not every patient will need a refeeding plan. Some eating disorder patients begin eating normally again once they receive initial attention and care. This decision is best made with the advice and input of a person's treatment team. Refeeding may elicit intense anxiety

Meal plan

A dietary guide that encourages adequate nutrition and caloric intake.

and nervousness in some patients; however, one's treatment team can assist in reducing concerns associated with weight gain. Relaxation exercises, psychotherapeutic techniques, and certain medications are just some of the tools that can help reduce any discomfort associated with refeeding.

Special Considerations

Severely malnourished patients will likely need a structured refeeding plan and generally call for a greater initial food intake than those who are better nourished. In order to maximize nourishment, nutritional supplements (such as Carnation Instant Breakfast, Ensure, or EnsurePlus) are often used as part of an initial food plan. Over time, supplements are reduced as nutritional balance is restored.

In severe cases, where marked dehydration, rapid weight loss, or significant electrolyte disturbance are manifest, emergency medical attention is given to refeeding. Universally, every attempt is made to elicit patient cooperation with refeeding; however, in rare cases, if food and nutrients are refused when a life-threatening risk is present, a medical team may implement compulsory refeeding. This can take place **intravenously** or with the use of a feeding tube, such as a **naso-gastric** tube (see Question 85 for more information). Artificial feeding is not preferred by doctors and is considered a last resort; thus, it is utilized only when medically necessary and is discontinued when it is no longer medically required. Additional medical circumstances (e.g., co-occurring diabetes mellitus) may be associated with a heightened risk of medical complications and may require hospitalization during the initial stages of weight restoration.

Intravenously

Injection of a substance or medication into a vein.

Naso-gastric

A tube that is inserted through the nose or mouth and into the stomach.

66. When I was struggling with my anorexia, I had a limited number of foods I would "allow" myself to eat. Can nutritional counseling help me learn to expand my food choices?

Yes! Both nutritional counseling and psychotherapy can be helpful tools for enabling you to expand the types of foods you eat, the range of food you purchase at the grocery store, and the variety of meals you prepare at home. A nutrition expert can also help you learn new skills for meal preparation and provide sample meal plans. (For sample meal plan suggestions, you can also visit *www.mypyramid.gov.*) Many patients avoid certain "feared foods" or may be used to eating pre-packaged "diet foods," leaving them with a limited range of natural, healthy foods to choose from. It can be a challenge to find variety for the three meals and two snacks per day that your doctor may recommend for you. (Note: Some prefer to eat 5–6 smaller meals throughout the day; you can discuss your preferences with your treatment team.) You also may be so used to reading nutrition labels and counting calories that the task of grocery shopping has become cumbersome. For practical help, I have offered some general recommendations for grocery shopping that may help you to expand your food choices while encouraging a healthy variety of nutrients in your regular diet.

Sample Grocery List

Fruit

- Apples, oranges, bananas, grapes, grapefruit, melon, strawberries, blueberries (fresh or canned)
- Fruit juice

Vegetables

- Potatoes, tomatoes, onions, green/red/yellow peppers, mushrooms, carrots, celery, cucumber, squash, zucchini, broccoli, cabbage (frozen, fresh, or canned)
- Garden burgers

Meats/proteins

- Hamburger, other lean beef, chicken breasts, turkey, fish
- Eggs
- Beans: pinto, white, navy, black (canned or dry versions)

Grains

- Whole grain bread for sandwiches and toast
- Hot or cold cereal, oatmeal, grits, waffles, pancake mix
- Brown rice, wild rice, pasta (assorted varieties)
- Bagels
- Tortillas
- Crackers
- Muffins or muffin mix

Dairy (good sources of calcium)

- Milk
- Yogurt (plain or flavored)
- Cottage cheese, cheese
- Frozen yogurt
- Carnation Instant Breakfast

Fats

- Peanut butter
- Margarine
- Nuts
- Mayonnaise
- Cream cheese

Desserts and snacks

- Cookies
- Brownies
- Cakes
- Ice cream
- Puddings
- Chips, pretzels, popcorn
- Granola

Other entrées

- Macaroni and cheese
- Spaghetti
- Pizza
- Chili
- Risotto
- Deli foods

Sarah shares:

I don't know if my eating disordered voices will ever disappear completely, or if I will ever look at food the way a "normal" person does. I've memorized the nutrition labels of every food in the grocery store, and that knowledge is hard to forget, especially now that the nutrition information is printed on foods even in restaurants.

But one of the most empowering feelings in the world is knowing exactly what is in the food I am eating, knowing that I once would have never let it get within 10 feet of my mouth, and eating it anyway, just because it tastes good. I can choose what I eat for entirely different reasons now.

67. How will my treatment team determine my healthy weight range?

Your therapist, physician, and nutrition counselor will gather information and use medical tests to evaluate an appropriate goal weight for your body type. Information that may be gathered includes: your eating disorder history and symptoms, highest and lowest past weights, alcohol and drug use, food preferences, food allergies, exercise habits, food associated with binge episodes, current eating patterns, and, in females, age at onset of menses and history of amenorrhea. Your doctor may take blood tests and measure your blood pressure, body temperature, and heart rate. Your healthy weight range will also take into account your height, age, body type, and activity level. An appropriate food plan will be determined based on all of these factors.

While it will be important to consume an adequate amount of food for weight restoration, many dietitians advise that patients in recovery avoid counting calories. Instead, they may recommend an approach that uses a food exchange system rather than calories as a guideline for weight restoration. Your treatment team can help you sort through the options and provide information to your family for informed decision making.

68. What changes should I expect in my body as I start to return to a healthy weight?

It may take some time to get used to healthy eating again.

It may take some time to get used to healthy eating again, however, your therapist and/or nutrition counselor will help you to feel increasingly comfortable with the process of weight restoration. You should be aware that in the initial stages of weight restoration, fluid retention is common as the body rehydrates itself. Therefore, you may notice some temporary swelling in your abdomen, face, thighs, and/or buttocks. **Delayed gastric emptying** is a frequent side effect of anorexia. Thus, you may feel bloated or experience abdominal pain after ingesting even small amounts of food. You should let your doctor know if these symptoms occur, as bloating may also be a sign of food allergies or food intolerance. Occasionally, patients in recovery report nighttime sweating or sweating after meals. This can result from changes to your metabolic rate due to increased food consumption.

Delayed gastric emptying

A decreased rate of emptying of the content in the stomach; also called gastroparesis. Delayed gastric emptying can cause nausea, vomiting, feeling full after a small meal, bloating, abdominal pain, and heartburn.

Interoceptive cues

Sensitivity to sensations that occur inside the body (e.g., gastrointestinal sensations, cardiac sensations).

You will be encouraged to eat at regular time intervals to help stabilize your metabolism and **interoceptive cues**. It may not be what you are used to, thus you may feel like you are eating "mechanically" at first. However, changes to your diet and food choices will take place gradually rather than all-at-once. Discuss your experiences, feelings, and thoughts with your treatment team. These caring professionals can help you work through any discomfort you may experience. It will be especially important to inform someone on your treatment team should you have the urge to binge, purge, or restrict your food intake. Remember that weight restoration is just

Weight restoration is just one part of the recovery process.

one part of the recovery process. Continue to work with your treatment team to ensure a complete recovery.

69. What is the Maudsley approach to weight restoration?

The Maudsley approach to weight recovery is based on a treatment method developed by two British researchers, Christopher Dare and Ivan Eisler, during the 1980s at the Maudsley Hospital in London. In the U.S., the approach has grown in popularity with the help of the book *How to Help Your Teenager Beat an Eating Disorder*. Long-term treatment outcomes appear to be promising. Studies show that children treated with the Maudsley approach recover faster and relapse less often. However, the approach is considered less effective for patients over the age of 18, or those who have prominent binge/purge symptoms, chronic illness, or families in which there is a high degree of interpersonal conflict.

In essence, the first priority of the Maudsley approach is regaining physical health and stability through refeeding. Unique to this approach is that it is the *parents* of an anorexia patient who lead the refeeding and healing process; a family therapist assists the parents in their efforts. After physical health is restored, emotional and social issues are addressed. According to the Maudsley Parents Web site (*http://maudsley parents.org*), there are three phases to treatment. First, parents are encouraged to normalize their child's eating while providing compassionate, non-judgmental support. A key intervention used during this phase includes the "coached family meal," a family-based meal that focuses on regaining control of a child's disordered eating, assisting with weight restoration, setting appropriate boundaries, and starting a patient on the road to recovery. In the second phase, once a patient's physical health is restored, the family works with a therapist to return control of eating to the recovering child. In the final phase of treatment, the focus shifts to helping the child establish a healthy adolescent identity. In this method, psychotherapy is not introduced into treatment until initial weight restoration is complete. For more information about the Maudsley approach, see the Resources section of this book.

70. Should I take a vitamin supplement when I am in recovery?

Individuals differ in their need for supplementation; however, anorexia patients are at increased risk for vitamin and mineral deficiencies. Your doctor may recommend supplementation of key vitamins and nutrients, but still, the best way to get them is through a balanced diet; merely taking supplements does not reduce the risk of complications that can arise from malnutrition. A balanced diet that includes a wide variety of foods can provide important vitamins, minerals, and other nutrients to patients in recovery. These include:

- **Vitamin A (beta-carotene):** Important for healthy eyes, skin, teeth, and immune functioning. Found naturally in fish and liver, and in certain fruits and vegetables.
- **Vitamin B complex:** Found in dairy products, meat, nuts, oatmeal, peanut butter, whole grains, yogurt, and some vegetables.
- **Vitamin B$_{12}$:** Found in beef, cheese, fish, eggs, liver, milk and milk products, pork, and tofu.
- **Vitamin C:** Found in green vegetables, berries and citrus fruits, mangos, sweet peppers, pineapple, radishes, spinach, and tomatoes.
- **Vitamin D:** Found in fish and dairy products fortified with Vitamin D, eggs, butter, milk, oatmeal, salmon, sardines, sweet potatoes, and tuna. With moderate amounts of exposure to sunlight, the body also naturally converts vitamin D. Both vitamin D and calcium are important in decreasing the risk of osteoporosis.
- **Vitamin E:** Found in vegetable oils, whole grains, nuts, seeds, peanuts, brown rice, eggs, milk, organ meats, sweet potatoes, soybeans, wheat germ, and dark-green, leafy vegetables.

- **Vitamin K:** Found in alfalfa, broccoli, soybeans, cauliflower, egg yolks, liver, oatmeal, rye, wheat, and dark-green, leafy vegetables.
- **Folic acid:** Found in beans, beef, whole grains, brown rice, cheese, chicken, dates, lamb, lentils, liver, milk, oranges, pork, salmon, tuna, yeast, and green, leafy vegetables. A deficiency of folic acid may contribute to depression and anxiety, and birth defects.
- **Calcium:** Found in dairy foods, seafood, seaweeds, nuts, buttermilk, cheese, shellfish, oats, parsley, prunes, whey, tofu, yogurt, and green, leafy vegetables. Calcium is an essential mineral for overall health and the prevention of osteoporosis. It should be combined with vitamin D for proper absorption.
- **Magnesium:** Found in most foods, especially dairy products, fish, meat, fruits, vegetables, whole grains, and seafood. The use of diuretics and laxatives, and purging behaviors can significantly contribute to magnesium deficiency.
- **Phosphorus:** Found in most foods, especially asparagus, bran, corn, dairy products, eggs, fish, dried fruit, garlic, sunflower and pumpkin seeds, meats, poultry, salmon, and whole grains. Important for electrolyte balance.
- **Potassium:** Found in dairy foods, fish, fruit, meat, poultry, vegetables, whole grains, dried fruit, garlic, lima beans, and nuts. Also important for electrolyte balance.
- **Sodium:** Found in most foods, but may need supplementation with use of laxatives, diuretics, or if purging symptoms are present. Important for electrolyte balance.
- **Zinc:** Found in fish, meats, poultry, seafood, egg yolks, lima beans, pecans, pumpkin seeds, soybeans, and whole grains. Some scientific studies have found zinc deficiencies in anorexia patients, suggesting that zinc may contribute to loss of appetite and affect a person's sense of taste and smell.
- **Iron:** Found in lean beef, prunes and other dried fruits, spinach, and whole grains.

- **Omega-3 fatty acids**: Found in fish oil, certain coldwater fish (e.g., salmon, herring, cod, and anchovies), cod liver oil, walnuts, and flax seeds. Essential fatty acids may play a critical role in brain function, heart function, and hormone regulation. Some studies also suggest that omega-3 fatty acids help to regulate mood and promote an anti-inflammatory response in the body.

71. Will I be able to stay on my vegetarian diet during recovery?

People with special dietary needs (e.g., vegetarians, vegans, those with reported food allergies or diabetes) should be sure to discuss dietary concerns with their physician and dietitian, as some special diets may increase the risk of vitamin and mineral deficiencies. In addition, be open with your treatment team about your reasons for following a special diet. While some people are vegetarians for religious or ethical reasons and some hold the belief that vegetarianism is a healthier way to eat (although there is little evidence to support this claim), special diets may also be a symptom of one's eating disorder. Distorted beliefs about food can hinder the recovery process; therefore, it is important to remain open about your dietary preferences and to discuss your unique needs with your treatment team.

72. What is orthorexia nervosa?

Introduced by Steven Bratman, orthorexia nervosa is a term used to describe a fixation with eating foods that are considered "pure" in quality. Literally translated, the term means "fixation on righteous eating." Although it is not an officially recognized medical condition, it can be a symptom of an eating disorder. Typical orthorexia behaviors include restricting foods to those perceived as "healthy," eating only organic foods, feeling guilty if "unapproved" foods are consumed, and self-punishing for deviations from these restrictions. Orthorexia can lead to social isolation, can impede healthy relationships, and may lead to physical and mental health problems. In contrast to anorexia, orthorexia is not necessarily associated with a desire to be thin or the fear of becoming fat. Thus, while it may be a contributing factor to anorexia or another eating disorder, its symptoms alone do not meet the criteria for anorexia nervosa.

73. A friend of mine was encouraged to keep a food diary when she was in treatment, but I find this worsens my tendency to obsess about food. Should I stop using the food diary?

Psychotherapists and nutritionists alike often recommend food diaries and food records when treating eating disorders. They are used to track progress in treatment, take note of disordered eating patterns, and identify antecedents to binge/purge behavior. However, studies show that for some patients, monitoring food intake is associated with an increase in eating disorders symptoms, food preoccupation, and body image dissatisfaction. This can be especially true with anorexia patients. In such instances, an alternative to a food diary is an "appetite diary." Appetite monitoring can help anorexia patients perceive physiological cues that signal hunger and **satiety**, something that is frequently impaired with an eating disorder. A typical diary entry may include the recognition of hunger cues (e.g., a gnawing feeling in the stomach, lightheadedness, stomach "growling," poor concentration, fatigue, headache, or an irritable mood) along with a hunger rating (e.g., on a scale of 1–10). Satiety cues are recorded in like manner. Appetite monitoring can also help patients distinguish between *physical* cues and *emotional* cues (such as anxiety, stress, shame, fear, anger) that may be mistaken for hunger or satiety—a problem that is common to eating disorder patients. Another alternative is a "food and feelings diary" in which a patient records his or her emotional reactions to mealtimes and food but does not include a record of the amount or types of foods eaten.

Satiety

The feeling of fullness or satisfaction after eating.

Lynn shares:

I'm sure there is much individual variation in how the issue of eating is experienced in people with anorexia. I was one who was constantly and ravenously hungry but afraid to eat. During this period, it was most helpful for me to concentrate on desired energy levels rather than track how much I was eating, which would have been overwhelming and frightening at that time. During times when I felt out of control and fearful of the weight gain, I would keep a record of the desired positive changes, such as improved ability to concentrate, improved sleep, better endurance, better performance, and feelings of increased strength and well-being.

74. I have always thought eating starchy foods would make me gain weight, but my dietitian says this is actually a "food myth." What are some other food myths?

Erroneous beliefs about food and weight gain are surprisingly common, even among the general population. However, inaccurate beliefs about food can lead to food aversions and may exacerbate eating disorders symptoms. Some of the most popularly held diet and food myths are listed here:

1. *Myth:* One extra snack will lead to immediate weight gain.
   Fact: For the average diet, it takes 3500 calories to gain one pound. Therefore, adding an extra snack will not cause immediate weight gain.

2. *Myth:* Dairy products cause weight gain.
   Fact: A certain *type* of food does not cause weight gain. Rather, weight gain is a function of total calories consumed, a person's energy expenditure, and metabolic rate.

3. *Myth:* Eating after 8 p.m. results in weight gain.
   Fact: See fact #2 of this list.

4. *Myth:* Red meat causes weight gain.
   Fact: See fact #2.

5. *Myth:* Fat-free foods do not cause weight gain.
   Fact: See fact #2.

6. *Myth:* Fried food goes straight to the hips and thighs.
   Fact: See fact #2.

7. *Myth:* If I eat more than my friends or family, it means I will get fat.
   Fact: See fact #2.

8. *Myth:* If I purge I will not be adding any calories for that meal.
   Fact: Experts note that most calories are retained despite self-induced vomiting or the use of laxatives.

9. *Myth:* Low-carbohydrate diets are good for you.
   Fact: Low-carbohydrate diets are not necessarily any better for you than a diet rich in complex carbohydrates. On the contrary, such diets may even be harmful. Low-carb diets may lead to fatigue, bone-loss, dehydration, hypoglycemia, mood imbalances, nutrient deficiencies, and electrolyte imbalances. Cholesterol levels and rate of blood flow to the heart can also be affected by diets that are extremely low in carbohydrates.

10. *Myth:* Eating certain foods in combination can cause weight loss or weight gain.
    Fact: The combining of foods has no effect on weight loss or weight gain.

11. *Myth:* Occasional fasting and "detox-diets" are good for your system.
    Fact: Recent research has shown that fasting has no impact on removing toxins from the body.

12. *Myth:* If I feel full, it means I have eaten too much.
    Fact: Satiety sensations do not indicate weight gain.

13. *Myth:* Some foods have weight-loss properties in them.
    Fact: Grapefruit, celery, and cabbage are examples of foods commonly referred to as "weight-loss foods" or "negative-calorie foods." There is no scientific evidence to support these claims.

14. ***Myth:*** Fat in a diet is bad for you.

    Fact: Fats are essential nutrients contained in food. Fats provide the body with energy and assist with satiety.

15. ***Myth:*** Sugar is addictive.

    Fact: In medical terms, sugar is not an addictive substance.

Lynn shares:

The myth that was scariest to me was that if I ate in accordance to hunger, my weight would continue to go up, and there would be no end to it. I also believed that all weight gain would of course be fat, and how could so many additional pounds of fat possibly be healthful? The truth is, when you gain weight after being severely underweight, there is a lot of lean body tissue mass added in addition to the essential fat reserves that account for weight gain.

PART NINE

Treatment and Recovery

How does a healthcare professional evaluate for anorexia?

How do I choose a treatment team?

What does treatment involve?

More . . .

75. How does a healthcare professional evaluate for anorexia?

A qualified healthcare professional will use a variety of assessment tools to establish an accurate diagnosis, assess for complications, and determine an appropriate course of treatment. An assessment can last anywhere from one hour to several office visits, depending on the complexity of the diagnostic picture. Frequently, a **multidisciplinary** team approach is used to provide a comprehensive assessment. For example, a qualified mental health professional may conduct a thorough **diagnostic interview** to establish a person's history of eating disorder symptoms, determine if symptoms meet the diagnostic criteria for an eating disorder, evaluate current stressors, and assess for any co-occurring psychiatric conditions. In addition, a physician will evaluate physical health status and assess the risk of physical complications. A dietitian may be called upon to evaluate nutritional needs and deficiencies. A comprehensive assessment may also include members of the patient's family, especially when the patient is still living at home, in order to provide collateral information, screen for a family history of eating disorders or other conditions, identify relevant family stressors, and provide the family with recovery support.

The treatment team may utilize a variety of professional tools during an evaluation. In addition to a clinical or diagnostic interview, healthcare professionals may use structured assessment instruments to assist with diagnosis and treatment planning. The Eating Disorder Examination, developed by Zafra Cooper and Christopher Fairburn, is one of the most widely used professional assessment instruments for eating disorders. Other popular assessment instruments are "self-report" in nature, meaning they are completed by patients and then returned to their treatment professionals, who incorporate the self-report data into the overall assessment and treatment plan. Self-report measures are used not only to help verify a clinical diagnosis, but also to help track changes

Multidisciplinary

Two or more professional disciplines working collaboratively. In health care, it refers to delivery of services by professionals from a variety of healthcare specialties.

Diagnostic interview

A structured or semi-structured interview of a patient, conducted by a healthcare professional in order to establish an accurate diagnosis of illness or condition.

in eating disorder symptoms over time. Examples of self-report measures include the Eating Disorder Inventory and the Eating Disorder Examination–Questionnaire. The most widely used self-report screening tool for eating disorders is the Eating Attitudes Test (EAT-26). The EAT-26 has been included in Appendix A for personal use. The EAT-26 alone is not designed to make a diagnosis of an eating disorder or to take the place of a professional diagnosis or consultation; *only a qualified healthcare professional can provide an accurate diagnosis.* However, the EAT-26 can be a first step in the screening process and can be useful for assessing eating disorder risk. (Note: All self-report measures require open and honest responses in order to gain accurate information. The fact that most people provide honest responses means the EAT-26 and other self-report measures usually offer very useful information about the eating symptoms and concerns common in eating disorders.)

76. What kinds of questions will I be asked during my assessment?

In the course of a comprehensive assessment, members of your treatment team will likely ask you most of the questions found in the following list. Keep in mind that your participation in any assessment interview is voluntary, and you can let your healthcare professional know if any of the questions make you uncomfortable, if you wish to return to a question later, or if you prefer not to answer. You have the right to feel comfortable with the assessment process as well as with the professional conducting the interview. By the same token, keep in mind that your treatment team will be able to take the best approach to your recovery when they are informed thoroughly about your history and symptoms.

Questions you may be asked include:

- Your age, marital status, and occupation
- Your education history

- Whether you have been in treatment before
- What concerns motivated you to seek help
- Dieting and weight history
- Your thoughts about food, eating, and weight gain
- Duration and intensity of eating disorder signs and symptoms
- Use of diet pills, laxatives, diuretics, or emetics
- Exercise patterns
- Your perceived body image
- Your developmental history
- Your general health history
- Your family's health history
- Any medications you take or allergies to any medications (including supplements)
- Your menstrual history (for females)
- Your energy level and sleep patterns
- Questions about your academic, social, occupational, and family functioning
- History of teasing or peer pressure
- Past or present drug or alcohol use
- Past or present physical, sexual, or emotional abuse
- Your personality, interests, and hobbies
- Questions to screen for anxiety, depression, suicidal thoughts/intent, and self-injurious behavior
- Questions to screen for other mental and physical disorders

If present, your family may be asked about family communication style, family relationships, general family history, your developmental history, and their observations of your eating disorder symptoms.

77. What kinds of laboratory tests will my physician conduct during assessment?

In addition to measuring your heart rate, blood pressure, and body temperature, your physician will want to conduct routine laboratory tests used to evaluate general physical health and may also want to screen for physical complications common to eating disorders. Laboratory tests may include:

- A basic blood analysis, which evaluates such things as electrolyte levels, **blood urea nitrogen (BUN), creatinine** level, blood glucose levels, and thyroid hormone level; this also provides a complete blood cell count (CBC), which checks for infection, anemia, and immune system functioning. Other markers of liver and kidney function can also be measured by a blood test.
- A urinalysis.
- An electrocardiograph (ECG), which records the electrical activity of the heart over time and is used to assess any abnormal rhythms of the heart muscle.
- Bone density tests.
- Hormone level assessments (for both males and females).
- Drug use screening, as indicated.
- Other tests as indicated, including pregnancy test, chest x-ray, heart stress test, and MRI.
- Additional tests may be required when symptoms of other physical illness or complications are present.

78. How do I choose a treatment team?

You may want to begin by asking for recommendations from friends, family, teachers, school counselors, members at your place of worship, your insurance carrier, or someone you know who has been in treatment. Your decisions may also depend on the level of care necessary in your particular situation (see Question 80). Resources such as the National Eating Disorders Association and the Web sites *www.edreferral.com* and *www.bulimia.com* offer helpful lists of treatment centers in locations across the United States. The Resources section of this book also includes a list of organizations that can provide resource listings in both the United States and Canada.

The relationships formed with your treatment team are an important part of the recovery process; therefore, it is

Blood urea nitrogen (BUN)

A blood test that helps to assess kidney function by measuring a waste product excreted by the kidneys.

Creatinine

A waste substance produced by the muscles. Measuring the creatinine level in the blood gives an indication of kidney functioning.

Treatment and Recovery

important that you feel comfortable with the professionals with whom you will be working. You have every right to ask questions and receive answers that will enable you to make an informed decision about whom you will select to assist with your recovery. Often, healthcare professionals are willing to answer some of your questions on the telephone, before establishing time for an initial consultation. Other questions can be answered in your initial face-to-face meeting, when the healthcare provider can become more familiar with you and your particular needs. A face-to-face consultation also allows you to observe the location and environment in which services will be provided.

Ideally, you will want to choose professionals experienced in treating anorexia. It is vital that the professionals be licensed or board certified in their respective fields of training. Professional and ethical behavior is necessary; if someone does not wish to answer your questions, seems distracted during your conversation, or is too busy to take the time to describe their services, you may wish to look elsewhere. You should feel that you can build working relationships with your caregivers, so choose people whose training and experience you can respect and who also communicate a sense of respect for *your* needs. Treatment is, in effect, a collaborative process, so the healthcare providers you select should appear willing to collaborate with you and your loved ones in the treatment process. Be aware of anything that may cause you initial discomfort when speaking to potential treatment providers; however, keep in mind that it may take time for a deeper sense of comfort and trust to develop.

You may wish to take this list of questions with you to your initial consultation, or keep it close by during your initial telephone call.

- What is your experience, and how long have you been treating eating disorders?
- Are you a licensed professional? What is your license type and number?

- Where did you receive your training?
- What type of treatment approach do you use?
- Do you use **evidence-based treatment** methods when treating eating disorders?
- What information do you use in formulating a treatment plan?
- How do you conduct your initial evaluation with patients?
- What other professionals will you be collaborating with for my treatment? Are they also familiar with eating disorders treatment?
- For therapists and dietitians: How is medical care integrated into your treatment approach? For physicians: How are psychotherapy and nutrition counseling integrated into your treatment approach?
- Do you involve family members in treatment?
- How do you maintain the confidentiality of my treatment records?
- What days and times do you have appointments available?
- How long do appointments last?
- How often will we meet for appointments?
- What is your fee for services? Do you accept insurance? What additional forms of payment do you accept?
- Do you offer a **sliding scale** fee structure?
- Do you have a Web site or any informational brochures that describe your services and background?
- What if I have questions or wish to contact you in between treatment sessions?
- Will I be able to reach you in the event of an emergency? If not, whom should I contact?

Additional questions to ask residential treatment facilities, partial hospital programs, or day-treatment programs:

- Do you offer travel assistance for patients who travel long distances to attend your program? Do you offer financial aid of any kind?

Evidence-based treatment

Treatment that seeks to apply the results of research evidence in establishing specific clinical guidelines for treatment effectiveness.

Treatment and Recovery

Sliding scale

A fee scale that fluctuates in response to a patient's income and cost-of-living.

- Do you offer any adjunct services for family members who wish to receive help?
- Is admission available now, or is there a waiting list?
- Are family members able to visit patients during treatment?
- How long is the average stay at your facility?
- Do you provide **aftercare** or offer a transitional program?
- What is the age range of patients at your facility?
- Is it a co-ed facility?
- Do you have experience with my special needs (e.g., adolescent patients, older patients, athletes, patients with a history of substance abuse)?
- What is the treatment philosophy followed at your facility?
- Do you use any alternative forms of therapy (e.g., art therapy, drama therapy)?
- How much time is devoted to group therapy and how much to individual therapy?
- Do you have a physician and nutrition counselor on staff?
- Can my family and I visit your facility before we make our decision?

Questions for families and loved ones to ask when needed:

- Do you recommend family therapy?
- If my child is in individual therapy, how often will you update me on his or her progress, and what information will you share with me regarding his or her treatment?
- What aspects of my child's treatment will remain confidential?
- Whom should I call if I have any questions about my child's treatment?
- Do you provide parent education and/or parent support groups? If not, can you recommend any for us?

Aftercare

Care services offered to a patient after he or she is discharged from a hospital or treatment program.

79. What kinds of professionals are included in a treatment team?

The most effective treatment team will be comprised of professionals from a variety of disciplines working together to comprehensively address the various aspects of recovery. The type and quantity of professionals included in the team will depend on factors such as severity of patient symptoms, level of care indicated, cost, location, and availability. Take care to select professionals with whom you are comfortable. In addition, you may need to go outside your local area for assistance if there are insufficient resources available in your region. Depending on the level of care needed, you may choose to start with one or two outpatient healthcare providers (i.e., a physician and therapist) and ask *them* to assist you in identifying other care providers in your area to add to your team. Do not feel like you need to go it alone in the recruitment and decision process. Treatment centers for patients who require a greater level of care (see Question 80) usually have a "built-in" team of staff already in place.

A comprehensive treatment team may include the following essential or non-essential individuals:

Essential:

- *A physician* who monitors and treats physical complications associated anorexia.
- *A mental health professional* who provides emotional support, helps to alleviate emotional distress, works to increase coping skills, assists with problem solving, and addresses various issues that contributed to the onset of the eating disorder and/or serve to maintain eating disorder symptoms. (See Exhibit 13 for more information about mental health professionals.)
- *A registered dietitian* who provides nutritional counseling and/or nutrition education.

Exhibit 13 Mental Health Providers

Mental Health Professional is a broad term that includes therapists from a variety of professional disciplines. License and credentialing requirements vary from state to state within the U.S., so check with your state's Consumer Affairs Department for more information. Education and training also varies among the different categories of therapists. For purposes of clarity, here is a description of the most popular categories of mental health professionals:

- *Psychologists* hold a doctorate degree in psychology (either a PhD, a PsyD, or an EdD). Four to seven years of training combines education in research, human behavior, assessment and diagnosis of mental illness, and a broad range of psychotherapeutic techniques. In the United States, psychologists are currently permitted to prescribe medication in a limited number of states.

- *Psychiatrists* are medical doctors with additional specialty training in mental health. Psychiatrists are able to prescribe medication.

- *Social workers* typically have a master's degree in social work (MSW or LCSW), which typically entails 2–4 years of education and training. Social workers may perform psychotherapy and may also offer skills training and assist with job placement or housing concerns.

- *Other therapists* may come from a variety of training backgrounds. Some hold a master's degree in a counseling-related field, such as marriage and family therapy, or psychiatric nursing. Others may not hold a master's degree but may have specialized training in particular areas, such as substance abuse. Each type of therapist or professional counselor has unique requirements for certification or licensure. Some of the letters you may see after the name of a master's level therapist or other counselor are LMFT, LMHC, LPC, and LPN.

Beneficial, when appropriate:

- *A physical therapist or exercise therapist* who helps determine appropriate levels of physical activity, and designs and supervises a balanced approach to physical activity and exercise.

- *A social worker* to help develop life skills necessary for independent living, such as cooking and food preparation, social skills, transportation, and housing.
- *Other medical professionals,* such as a dentist who can evaluate any adverse effects on oral health brought about by purging and a gynecologist or endocrinologist who can evaluate and treat hormonal imbalances that may have resulted from an eating disorder.

Optional but desirable:

- *Psychopharmacologist* when necessary, to evaluate medications that may assist with recovery (may or may not be the chosen physician). State provisions vary, but prescribing providers may include physicians, clinical nurse practitioners, and psychologists.
- *Experiential therapist* who can incorporate various adjunct therapies when appropriate and desired, such as art therapy, music therapy, yoga, massage therapy, drama therapy, and equine therapy.
- *Coaches, teachers, and friends* who can provide needed support and encouragement.
- *Paraprofessional or peer support group facilitators* who can provide a forum for shared experiences, assertiveness and social skills training, and social support.

80. What is meant by "level of care," and how does it affect my treatment options?

Level of care refers to the intensity of treatment determined for a patient, given their symptoms and risk for complications. Five basic levels of care are utilized in eating disorders treatment (see Exhibit 14 for a summary of level of care guidelines). Additional factors such as medical risk, body weight, comorbid conditions, and motivation for recovery are considered when determining the most appropriate level of patient care.

Treatment and Recovery

Exhibit 14 Summary of Guidelines for Determining the Appropriate Level of Patient Care

Inpatient Hospitalization

Medically unstable:

- Acute health risk
- Weight <85% of normal range
- Acute weight decline with food refusal

Psychiatrically unstable:

- Rapidly worsening symptoms
- Moderate to high risk for suicide
- Co-occurring psychiatric disorder that may require hospitalization
- Needs supervision during and after all meals or needs special feeding

Residential Treatment

Medically stable:

- No intensive medical intervention needed
- Weight generally <85% of normal range

Psychiatric impairment:

- Needs supervision to gain weight and to prevent excessive exercise
- Inadequate social support
- May show moderate risk for suicide

Partial Hospitalization

Medically stable:

- No immediate risk

Psychiatrically stable, however:

- Needs some structure to assist with weight gain and to prevent excessive exercise

Intensive Outpatient or Outpatient

Medically stable, psychiatrically stable, and:

- Has sufficient social and/or familial support
- Adequate skills for self-sufficiency

SOURCE: American Psychiatric Association. (2006). *Practice guideline for the treatment of patients with eating disorders*, 3rd ed. Washington, DC: Author.

The five basic levels of care for eating disorders treatment are as follows:

1. *Outpatient care*: A patient meets with one or more treatment providers one to three times per week in an office setting. Sessions typically last 45 minutes to an hour. Outpatient care is generally provided by collaboration between a physician, psychotherapist, and registered dietitian.

2. *Intensive outpatient care (IOP)*: A patient attends a treatment program several days each week, full or half days. This option allows for increased structure, support, education, and monitoring. Additional therapeutic activities and some meals are provided. The patient sleeps at home at night.

3. *Partial hospitalization care* (also known as full-day treatment): Similar to an IOP program, but a patient generally attends 5 full days per week, 4–8 hours per day. All daytime meals are provided. Nutritional and medical needs are closely monitored. This method provides greater structure and patient accountability. The patient sleeps at home at night.

4. *Residential treatment facility (RTF) care*: A patient lives at a facility that offers extended care (usually no longer than 6 months), including group and individual psychotherapy, medical and nutritional monitoring, patient education, and alternative therapies. Residential treatment facilities are intended to be a home-like setting where patients can practice the coping skills they learn in therapy sessions while they are in a structured, supervised program. Residential treatment is not intended for patients who have acute medical or psychiatric symptoms. Length of stay and cost vary.

5. *Inpatient hospitalization* (also known as medically managed, or intensive treatment): A patient is treated in a hospital setting because they require 24-hour medical monitoring due to medical risk or complications, or other immediate risk. Length of stay can vary from a few hours to a week or more.

81. What does treatment involve?

In the following paragraphs, I highlight three important aspects of successful anorexia treatment.

First, treatment involves comprehensive care. The most effective treatment for anorexia involves a comprehensive, team-based approach that addresses, at a minimum, mental health, medical health, and nutritional care. Studies show that a multidisciplinary approach, which may include a variety of therapies (see Figure 8), is associated with enhanced treatment effectiveness and yields the best treatment outcomes. While individualized treatment plans vary, aspects of a comprehensive approach to treatment may include:

- Individual psychotherapy: A trained psychotherapist meets one-on-one with a patient and provides mental health care intended to ameliorate eating disorders symptoms through behavior change. Psychotherapy helps to promote flexible and adaptive thinking, increase coping skills, and address emotional and relational issues that may be affecting health and well-being.
- Group psychotherapy: Patients meet in a group setting with one or more therapists. The modality of group therapy will vary based on the facilitator's approach: Some will utilize "talk-therapy," some will be **didactic**, and others may incorporate experiential therapies such as art, music, or drama. Skills-based groups offer training in assertiveness, coping skills, social skills, interpersonal skills, and distress tolerance. Group therapy provides an increased sense of social support and offers an environment in which group members can relate to shared experiences. Paraprofessionally facilitated "support groups" are another option. To maximize the benefit of group therapy, care is taken to avoid "triggering" topics of discussion (such as weight-loss techniques and purging methods).

Didactic

Intending to instruct or educate.

- Family therapy: Interventions geared toward maximizing family cohesion and reducing family stress help to improve patient support. Family support and didactic groups are also available.
- Nutrition counseling (see Question 61).
- Medication, as needed (see Question 90).
- Ongoing medical attention, as indicated.
- Adjunct support from significant others, including friends, teachers, clergy, and coaches.

Second, treatment involves commitment. The importance of committing to the recovery process cannot be overemphasized. Early treatment dropout has been shown to adversely affect prognosis for recovery; yet nearly one-third of anorexia patients end treatment prematurely, leading to a relapse of symptoms. Perhaps the most important piece of advice you will receive is to *STICK WITH TREATMENT.* Your treatment team can help you work through any discouragements, doubts, fears, or lapses in motivation that may arise.

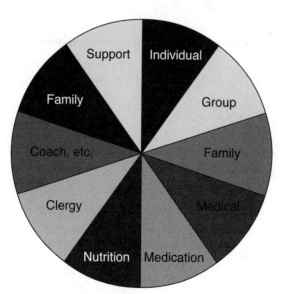

Figure 8   A Comprehensive, Multidisciplinary Approach to Treating Anorexia Nervosa

Treatment and Recovery

*Recovery
is a process
that involves
changes over
time.*

Third, treatment involves a process. Recovery is a process that involves changes over time and includes its share of difficulties; however, that is to be expected. In any healing process, some changes will occur more gradually than others. Yet it is not just in the *measurable* changes that recovery takes place. Recovery also takes place in the *process of growth and change*— the self-discovery that leads to a greater sense of completeness, empowerment, and well-being. Lindsey Hall and Monika Ostroff, authors of *Anorexia Nervosa: A Guide to Recovery*, share personal insights from their own journeys of healing with these words: "Recovery is a process, not an event. It is unique to each person, but in every case demands commitment, determination, and willingness. Recovery obliges you to open up, to discover and share parts of yourself, and to connect with the people in your life." Hall and Ostroff elaborate:

> In the beginning stages, the tendency is to believe that recovery means achieving and maintaining a certain weight. However, as recovery unfolds, the attention shifts inward ... leading to a deeper and more meaningful understanding of one's self and one's place in the world. The path of recovery is inescapably sprinkled with frustrating setbacks and plateaus that at times may cause you to wonder if you are moving forward. However, these times are actually tremendous opportunities to learn.

There is no "perfect" path to recovery. In truth, the road may include its share of bumps, detours, and unexpected turns. That is the nature of recovery, and, in fact, part of the human experience. Gaining a greater understanding of our vulnerabilities as well as our strengths is part of the complete recovery landscape, a picture that includes greater authenticity, self-care, self-acceptance, perspective, empowerment, and peace. And as Hall and Ostroff have aptly described, even the difficult challenges associated with recovery bring their share of learning and personal reward.

82. How long does recovery take?

That can be difficult to say because the time will vary from person to person. Studies show that a patient's age, duration of symptoms, severity of symptoms, and the presence of certain co-occurring conditions can affect treatment duration. Additionally, patients with a lower body weight at the time of treatment tend to have a longer path toward recovery than those closer to a normal weight. Studies indicate recovery from anorexia takes an average of 5 to 7 years. May it take you less time? Will it take longer? You may not know at the outset of treatment, but you may get a better indication as healing begins to take place. Is it worth taking steps toward recovery even if you do not know how long it will take? *Yes!* Recovery is *absolutely* worth the time and effort—however long it takes.

Lynn shares:

When I heard that recovery was discussed in the time frame of years, I felt rather depressed and anxious. However, I was envisioning some sort of torturous struggle, similar to what I was experiencing in the disease. Once you commit yourself to recovery and have a team in place to help you through it, there is a huge sense of relief.

Recovery work is hard and scary, but it can also be fun and enlightening. One of the most healing times I had involved some evening discussions with a friend who was recovering from an alcohol addiction. We compared experiences and recovery paths and found we could see new perspectives together that we never saw on our own. We could even really laugh at ourselves, which was enormously healing and fun. Yes, there is a lot in recovery that is fun, and there are opportunities for growth and self-learning that you would have never encountered otherwise. You learn a deeper understanding of and empathy for the struggles of others. You come out of the disorder with skills, strengths, and life experiences that allow you to embrace the past difficulties with a sort of gratitude.

Treatment and Recovery

Recovery is absolutely worth the time and effort— however long it takes.

I believe the process of recovery never really ends because I see it as the process of continuing growth as an individual. As the symptoms of the eating disorder fade away, you continue in a new life that is more meaningful, fun, and enjoyable as time goes on.

Sarah shares:

Physically, I recovered almost entirely during my time in treatment. With the help of professionals whom I trusted and who cared for me, I was able to get back to a healthy weight in a matter of months.

My mental recovery, however, took a little bit longer. When it came down to it, I felt like the food I put in my mouth was one of the few things I had true control over. This is why anorexia (or any eating disorder) is such a powerful sickness. It took me a long time to recognize my eating disorder as a separate entity within myself, but once I did, it was a lot easier to deal with parting with it. I learned that my eating disorder didn't define me and that I could in fact live a much happier life without it. Four years later, I still work every day to remain separate from my eating disorder, but aside from the occasional bump in the road, every day I am getting stronger and stronger.

83. How will I know when I am getting better?

According to the treatment guidelines established by the American Psychiatric Association, goals targeted for recovery from anorexia include:

- Medical and physical stability
- Normalized eating
- Normalized levels of physical activity
- Increased patient understanding about eating disorders
- The absence of purging
- Increased psychological coping mechanisms
- Treatment of co-occurring issues or conditions
- Enhanced social and interpersonal functioning

Recovery markers for these treatment goals include normal laboratory data, a return to a healthy weight, reduced risk of suicide or self-harm, decreased eating disordered behaviors, reduced body image disturbance, improved interaction with family and friends, and a realistic plan to avoid relapse.

In addition, many eating disorder specialists assert that complete recovery from anorexia includes improvements not addressed by the aforementioned treatment guidelines. Of interest to these experts are *subjective* improvements in functioning, such as hopefulness, personal empowerment, identity, and inner peace. There is, however, a lack of consensus as to which such elements constitute "a full recovery." Toward that end, psychologists Dan Reiff and Kathleen Kim Lampson Reiff have developed a helpful list of suggested "personal indicators of recovery." Included in Exhibit 15 is a revised and abbreviated version of this list. Keep in mind as you review it that there is no "perfect recovery." Instead, the ultimate recovery goal is a healthy, well-balanced life that consists of emotional, physical, social, and relational balance. The recovery markers presented are intended to encourage this goal.

Lynn shares:

The most important indicator of recovery for me was the amazing increase in life enjoyment. I no longer just endured the day; I actually enjoyed it. My focus could be on things other than what I did or didn't eat and how that might affect me. I was able to concentrate on work, relationships, and new skills, and could actually be fully present for them. I felt increasingly healthy and alive, with improved strength and endurance, and wanted to continue on this course. These feelings would be interspersed with times of stress when I questioned everything I was doing and felt the familiar fears and despair associated with the anorexia. There is the tendency to believe that one day or period of falling back will cancel out all the days of progress. It isn't true. One of the stumbling blocks to recovery is thinking that it has to be done perfectly. It won't be that way, and understanding and accepting that is in itself a part of

Treatment and Recovery

Exhibit 15   Psychological, Relational, and Emotional Indicators of Recovery

Indicators of recovery regarding self:

- Self-esteem: learning to base self-worth on who you are on the "inside."
- Perfectionism: recognizing and accepting imperfection in yourself and others.
- Support network: developing a broad-based network of people to turn to for emotional support.
- Validation of feelings: learning to accept and validate your own feelings as well as the feelings of others.
- Responsibility: accepting age-appropriate responsibility for making your recovery and your life what you want them to be.
- Approval: increased ability to withstand the disapproval or disagreement of others.
- Guilt: learning to distinguish between appropriate and inappropriate guilt.
- Pleasure: increasing relaxation, spontaneity, humor, and joy.
- Sexuality: facing any fears concerning sexuality and learning how to establish boundaries with oneself and others in sexual relationships.
- Body image: accepting your body the way it looks when you are maintaining a healthy weight.
- Identity: learning to find and develop passionate pursuits in life other than and apart from weight, shape, and appearance.
- Assertiveness: learning to express your feelings, desires, and opinions to others.

Indicator of recovery regarding family:

- Family limitations: recognizing your family's limitations and learning healthy ways of interacting with family members.

Indicators of recovery regarding relationships:

- Emotions: learning to identify and respond to emotional states including grief, loss, anger, sadness, and disappointment; learning to express feelings in a way that promotes emotional closeness with others rather than emotional distance; learning to resolve conflict in a healthy way.
- Intimacy and trust: building and maintaining intimate relationships that are loving, collaborative, and open.
- Interdependence: learning to build interdependent relationships in which needs are clearly communicated and appropriate limits are set.

SOURCE: Reiff, D. W., and Lampson Reiff, K. K. (1997). *Eating disorders: Nutrition therapy in the recovery process.* (pp. 466–467). Mercer Island, WA: Life Enterprises Publications. (help@ eatingdisorderssupport.com)

recovery. You just ride through the tough days and keep on going, finding that the feelings of life enjoyment and freedom from the eating disorder get stronger and more frequent as the anorexia fades away.

Sarah shares:

Every so often I'll wake up in the morning and eat pancakes for breakfast, or get out of bed and realize I really don't want to run. Or I'll go out to eat at a restaurant I never once would have gone to, at a time that once would have been off-limits. Most of the time, I do these things without even realizing how many former "rules" I'm breaking. It's the little things like this that let me know just how much I have let go of my anorexia; and knowing that I no longer need my eating disorder is the most rewarding feeling in the world.

84. What is "transition care," and how important is it to eating disorder treatment?

Transition care (also known as transition-phase treatment) refers to the preparation and training provided to patients who will soon leave inpatient or residential treatment. Transition care includes such practical concerns as helping patients to coordinate a follow-up treatment team in their home region as well as determining what tangible needs patients may have upon their return home. Emotional preparation for transitioning back into daily life is another important component of transition care. Transition programs also provide patients with an opportunity to gain confidence as they practice newly acquired coping skills. Studies show that patients find transition care extremely helpful in the overall course of recovery.

Treatment and Recovery

85. What can be done if a person with anorexia is in critical danger but still refuses treatment?

Ideally, patients will express a commitment to beginning the recovery process *or at least* will be willing to explore the option of receiving treatment when they feel they are ready. However, some people with a suspected eating disorder may resist the idea of seeking treatment, and there may be occasions when a medical doctor may consider imposing treatment against a patient's stated wish. Such cases arise when there is a decidedly imminent threat to a person's life due to either medical complications or extreme risk for suicide. Referred to as "involuntary treatment" or "compulsory treatment," this type of intervention can involve confining a person to a treatment facility (e.g., a hospital) and/or imposing involuntary feeding, such as with the use of a naso-gastric feeding tube. Healthcare professionals express conflicting opinions about the use of involuntary treatment. Most, however, believe it should only be undertaken as a last resort. Indeed, in the past, the benefits of involuntary treatment were considered dubious. Recently, however, research has suggested that compulsory treatment may be just as effective in the short term as voluntary treatment. Long-term effects of involuntary treatment have yet to be discovered, but research is currently underway.

86. What are some of the psychological treatments currently used for treating anorexia?

A number of distinct psychotherapy approaches are currently in use. Variables such as the training of the therapist, the age and background of the patient, the setting for treatment (hospital versus outpatient, for example), and symptom severity all influence the application of the various psychotherapies. There is little empirical data with regard to the comparative effectiveness of psychological treatments for anorexia. Indeed, a majority of therapists choose to integrate multiple therapies in treatment, rather than adhere to a singular approach. This is a practice known as "eclectic" or "integrative" therapy. The following is a brief description of some of the most commonly utilized treatments.

- ***Cognitive-behavioral therapy*** (CBT) is the most frequently studied individual psychotherapy treatment for anorexia nervosa. It postulates an interconnectedness between a person's thoughts, feelings, and behaviors. The approach asserts that the way a person *thinks* will affect the way that person *feels* and *behaves* (the interactions between these three factors is conceptualized in Figure 9). CBT, in part, seeks to correct maladaptive thought patterns that may influence eating disorders symptoms, thereby helping to reduce unhealthy behaviors. It also seeks to enhance skills for coping with stress and anxiety. CBT includes aspects of "talk therapy" and frequently incorporates "homework" exercises geared toward supporting and enhancing positive change. Education about eating disorders is also included in CBT treatment. CBT is considered one of the most effective treatments for bulimia nervosa, so it is not surprising that it is a frequent choice for anorexia patients. However, issues such as symptom severity, motivation, treatment setting, duration of treatment, and medical risk may affect the usefulness of CBT with some anorexia patients.

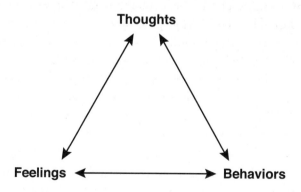

Figure 9   The Relationship Between Thoughts, Feelings, and Behaviors (as conceptualized in Cognitive-Behavioral Therapy)

- *Family therapy* is considered a standard approach to the treatment of anorexia in adolescents and has also been used successfully with adult patients. It is the most extensively researched treatment for anorexia, and the results thus far have been encouraging. Family therapy may include didactic education about eating disorders, improving family relationships, clarifying individual roles within the family, reducing family conflict, improving communication, and providing patient and family support. Individual psychotherapy may be used in conjunction with a family therapy approach.

- *Behavioral therapies* are those most frequently used to promote weight gain in severely malnourished patients. For example, reinforcing adaptive and healthy behaviors through reward is a longstanding technique used in the weight restoration phase of eating disorders treatment. Behavioral therapies can be combined with, or replaced by, other psychotherapy approaches as cognitive functioning improves and a patient's weight is restored.

- *Psychodynamic psychotherapy* is a popular approach for a broad range of mental health concerns. It seeks to address the underlying issues related to emotional distress, increase self-awareness, and resolve underlying psychological conflicts. This approach frequently explores a person's past to bring greater insight into one's present behavior. The benefits of this approach are found in a strong emphasis on the therapist–patient relationship. Research into the effectiveness of psychodynamic therapies with anorexia is growing in number, but still limited (Zerbe 2007). Some experts caution that psychodynamic psychotherapies are not recommended for patients in a weakened physical state, those who have difficulty identifying and expressing their feelings, or those with a reduced distress tolerance.

- *Interpersonal therapy* (IPT) underscores the importance of significant relationships and social functioning in recovery. It is a short-term treatment approach that has been proven effective in the treatment of depression and eating disorders and may also be integrated into longer-term treatment of anorexia.

- *Feminist therapy* focuses on the cultural context of eating disorders. It seeks to address the way gender roles, identity confusion, and trauma affect one's psychological well-being. Among its many facets, this approach incorporates assertiveness training, relationship building, and personal empowerment.

- *Dialectical behavior therapy* (DBT) is a contemporary therapy that was developed by psychologist Marsha Linehan as an extension of traditional CBT methods. It incorporates teachings about **mindfulness** and acceptance while concurrently promoting behavior change. It was developed for use with complex mental illnesses and has demonstrated empirical success in treating suicidal behaviors and self-injury. More recently, DBT has been introduced as a helpful approach for treating eating disorders. DBT integrates skills training in areas such as distress tolerance, interpersonal effectiveness, and emotional regulation in order to help patients modify extreme behaviors so they may become more balanced.

- *Non-specific supportive clinical management* (SCM) is an approach that couples clinical management of anorexia symptoms with psychological support that does not strictly adhere to one form of therapy over another. However, SCM includes some qualities that are central to a number of modalities, including unconditional acceptance of the patient, empathic understanding, and positive regard. The primary focus of this approach is the resumption of normal eating and the restoration of weight; however, other life issues that may impact eating disorder symptoms are also addressed.

- *Experiential therapies and alternative therapies* are frequently used in conjunction with more structured therapeutic techniques and may be incorporated into a broader approach to treatment. Various new therapies are under investigation, including *cognitive remediation therapy*, which uses cognitive exercises to help patients

Mindfulness

A moment-to-moment awareness of one's thoughts, feelings, motivations, and actions. Mindfulness originated as a state of meditation within the Buddhist tradition.

Treatment and Recovery

strengthen their thinking skills and demonstrate increased cognitive flexibility. Experiential activities such as art therapy and play therapy allow children and adolescents to express their feelings through non-verbal methods. Relaxation therapy teaches techniques to reduce stress, and body image therapy seeks to improve patient self-perception of body image. Spiritual approaches to recovery can be incorporated in keeping with patient preferences. Meditation, yoga, drama therapy, creative writing, movement therapy, **hypnotherapy**, and music therapy are other examples of alternative therapies occasionally used in anorexia recovery.

Hypnotherapy

The use of hypnosis in therapy. In hypnotherapy, a patient is guided to a state of focused relaxation to facilitate behavioral, emotional, or attitudinal change.

87. What is "motivational interviewing," and how can it help with recovery?

Motivational interviewing (MI), also called "motivational enhancement therapy," is a collaborative technique that seeks to understand a person's level of readiness and motivation for recovery while engaging their active participation in identifying goals for change. Some of the most popular psychotherapies were developed for use with motivated adults. However, these approaches may not be as effective with patients who lack the personal motivation needed for recovery. MI seeks to address these motivational concerns so that even patients with a great deal of resistance may benefit. Toward that end, MI avoids direct persuasion and instead harnesses each patient's unique level of readiness in order to support change.

MI grew from the work of Drs. James Prochaska, Carlo DiClemente, and John Norcross, whose efforts identified multiple "stages of change" that people encounter when they attempt to work through a problem. These stages reflect the level of motivation people may experience as they think about changing problematic behaviors. MI seeks to understand and apply these stages of change on an individual basis to help patients explore their own ambivalence about recovery and move through the stages toward a positive outcome. From their research, the following five stages of change were identified:

1. *The Precontemplation Stage*: a person may not be aware they have a problem, may deny their problem, or may express an unwillingness to change.
2. *The Contemplation Stage*: a person may be thinking about change, but he or she may be fearful of change or remain unconvinced help is needed.
3. *The Preparation Stage*: a person intends to change and makes a commitment to do so, even if they are unsure what steps to take.
4. *The Action Stage*: a person takes tangible steps toward change.
5. *The Maintenance Stage*: a person practices newly acquired behaviors and takes steps to prevent relapse.

88. My therapist and my dietitian both use the term "cognitive distortions" when they talk about my eating disorder symptoms. Can you explain what these are and how they may be affecting me?

"Cognitive distortion" is a term associated with cognitive-behavioral therapy (CBT). It refers to a *biased way of thinking* about oneself or one's environment, including one's body image, weight, or appearance—namely, the kinds of biases that can exacerbate anorexia symptoms. Therapists who are CBT oriented work with patients to modify and eliminate these kinds of thinking errors. Cognitive distortions are extremely common among eating disorder patients, as well as among people who experience anxiety and depression. Do you recognize any of the following cognitive distortions in your own thinking?

- *"All or nothing thinking"*—extremes in thinking. For example, things are either *good* or *bad, black* or *white*; there is no in between. ("I am a failure because I ate too much today.")

- *Over-generalizing*—drawing global conclusions from a single, isolated event. ("He is late again. I *always* have to be the responsible one in the family.")
- *Catastrophizing*—assuming and expecting the worst in a given situation. ("If I binge again, I have no hope of getting better.")
- *Mind reading*—assuming what other people are thinking or feeling without asking them. ("She thinks I'm lazy.")
- *Personalizing*—assuming that someone else's behavior was in reaction to you and/or assuming responsibility for those actions. ("He went out with his friends because he thinks I'm dull.")
- *Self-fulfilling prophecy*—expecting an outcome before it occurs, thereby increasing the likelihood of it happening. ("I always binge before work.")
- *"What-if's"*—asking yourself "what-if" questions that lead you to worry and focus on negative possibilities and outcomes. ("What if there is nothing at the restaurant I can eat?")
- *The "shoulds," "musts," and "have-tos"*—having unbending rules for oneself. ("I *should not* eat that other cookie," or "I *have to* be the one who gets straight A's.")
- *Superstitious or magical thinking*—irrational attributions to oneself or the world. ("I am not allowed to be happy.")
- *Emotional reasoning*—making judgments based on feelings, not on facts. ("I hate it when my son cries. I am a terrible mother.")
- *Comparisons*—judging oneself in comparison to others. ("She didn't finish her plate; she must have more willpower than I do.")

89. How can assertiveness training help with recovery?

Assertiveness involves speaking up for one's own feelings and needs—something that is characteristically very difficult for someone with an eating disorder. Recall that many anorexia patients also have difficulty identifying and expressing feelings or asking for help. Instead, anorexia becomes the non-verbal "voice" patients use to let others know about their emotional pain, personal challenges, and needs that might otherwise go unexpressed. After all, anorexia has a way of poignantly saying, "Leave me alone," or "Back off!" or "I just wish I could disappear." Moreover, individuals accustomed to *distracting, soothing,* or *avoiding* their feelings with exercise, binging, purging, or restricting calories, may find it intimidating and unsettling to imagine getting in touch with those feelings they have been desperately trying to avoid. Yet, learning to comfortably express one's own opinions, thoughts, and feelings can provide significant help along the road to recovery. This is where assertiveness training comes in. Assertiveness training is a straightforward process of learning how to become more comfortable expressing one's own feelings, reactions, wants, and needs to others. Studies show that assertiveness training can help build confidence, assist with managing stress and anger, and improve coping skills for emotional health and well-being.

Many anorexia patients have difficulty identifying and expressing feelings or asking for help.

Would you benefit from assertiveness training? Complete the following statements by answering with:

(A) Always (B) Frequently (C) Sometimes (D) Rarely (E) Never

1. I stand up for my own needs.
2. I feel I deserve to be heard.
3. I believe I have a right to my own feelings and opinions.
4. I share my feelings and opinions with others.
5. I ask for what I want and need.
6. I am able to say "no" when I do not want to do something.

Treatment and Recovery

7. I am afraid it will seem selfish if I express my feelings or opinions.

If you answered C, D, or E to most of questions 1–6, and/or answered A or B to question 7, you will likely benefit from assertiveness training.

The following are some useful strategies involved in assertiveness training. You may want to practice with your treatment team or a trusted friend to build your confidence. Being assertive takes time and practice. Your skill and ease will increase over time, so be patient with yourself.

- Use assertive language. Use "I" statements so that others know what you are thinking and feeling. For example, instead of saying, "You are ignoring me!" you could say, "I feel hurt when you watch television when I'm trying to speak to you." (See Question 55 for more about "I" statements.)
- Be clear in asking for what you want. For example, if you are going to the movies and picking up a friend who has a reputation for being late, you could say, "I really want to get there for the previews, so please be ready to go at 7 o'clock."
- Speak up if you are overlooked. For example, if you are waiting in line at the grocery store and someone steps in front of you, it is okay to say, "Excuse me, I'm not sure if you saw me, but I was in line ahead of you."
- Do not apologize for your feelings. Do not apologize when you have not done anything wrong.
- Do not take responsibility for someone else's behavior.
- Repeat your request, if you are not satisfied that you have been heard.
- Express yourself calmly, taking deep breaths if you need to. Avoid insults and accusations. For example, instead of saying, "You are so stubborn, you *never* listen to me!" you could say, "I feel frustrated when you interrupt me, so please just listen for a moment."

- Listen to others' points of view as well—but remember that you do not have to agree with their opinion or do what they are asking.
- Offer to compromise, when appropriate.

90. Are there any medications that help with anorexia?

Perhaps it goes without saying, but the VERY BEST medicine for anorexia is FOOD. Remember, many of the symptoms associated with anorexia are a direct result of starvation. Therefore, adequate nutrition and weight restoration are key elements for symptom reduction and recovery.

To date, the evidence base for the use of medication for anorexia has yielded few positive results. Furthermore, studies show that medication in the absence of psychotherapy is ineffective and contraindicated for anorexia patients. There are currently no medications approved by the FDA for the purpose of weight restoration from anorexia. In terms of **off-label use**, clinical studies have shown that two **psychotropic** medications reveal a *moderate* benefit with weight restoration: olanzapine (also called Zyprexa) and quetiapine (also called Seroquel). Both olanzapine and quetiapine belong to a class of medications known as "atypical antipsychotics." These medications are primarily used to treat thought disorders, severe mood disorders, delusions, and hallucinations; yet clinicians find that these medications may help some anorexia patients by reducing eating disorder symptoms, obsessions, agitation, and anxiety. Some studies show that these medications may help anorexia patients better appreciate the severity of their condition and engage in treatment (Mickley 2004). While there is not yet *definitive* evidence of the effectiveness of these medications on weight gain, further study is underway. Additional atypical antipsychotic medications are also under investigation for their effects on anorexia symptom reduction and weight gain.

Off-label use

The permissible use of a drug in ways other than what was originally sanctioned.

Psychotropic

A medication or agent that affects mental functioning or behavior.

Clinical trials have also investigated the use of a class of antidepressants known as selective serotonin re-uptake inhibitors (SSRIs) in the treatment of eating disorders. You may recognize some of their common names: Paxil, Prozac, Zoloft, Lexapro, and Celexa. Although these medications are helpful with some aspects of eating disorders recovery in normal-weight patients, none of these medications has been found helpful in the weight restoration phase of anorexia recovery. However, studies have found that some SSRIs may be useful for some patients once they have returned to and sustained a normal weight. SSRIs may help to reduce symptoms of depression and anxiety, and may also reduce other unwanted symptoms, such as obsessions and binge behaviors. Another class of antidepressant, known as tricyclic antidepressants, has been associated in controlled studies with faster weight gain and improved mood for anorexia patients. Other studies point to possible benefits from the time-limited use of certain anti-anxiety medications for help with anorexia recovery. In addition, anorexia patients may benefit from medications that address symptoms of co-occurring conditions, such as mood disorders and ADHD.

If your doctor recommends medication as a part of your treatment, be sure to follow his or her recommendations very carefully. Some medications can be habit forming and should be used with caution in patients with a history of substance abuse. Other medications (for example, the mood stabilizer lithium) should be used with caution in anorexia patients. As with any medication, closely monitor any changes that take place, and inform your family physician if you notice side effects such as heart arrhythmia, an increase in eating disorder symptoms, changes in mood, or an increase in suicidal thoughts.

91. What should I know about the confidentiality of my child's discussions in psychotherapy?

Confidentiality, or the right to patient privacy, is an important aspect of treatment. Recovery may involve sharing very delicate feelings and personal thoughts that a patient may not wish to have shared with others; therefore, every patient will want to have an informed discussion with his or her therapist about confidentiality. This is especially true as it applies to adolescent patients and their parents. While parents of non-**emancipated**, minor children have the legal right to their children's patient health information, young people may feel more comfortable sharing their thoughts when they know this information will remain private. Parents and their children should discuss concerns about confidentiality with their caregivers at the outset of treatment so everyone involved is informed and can feel comfortable with the level of privacy established. Privacy of conversations does not mean parents cannot be involved in a child's treatment; indeed, they should be involved. Patients are encouraged to share information with their parents when it is in their best interest to do so. In addition, if patients become at risk for serious harm to themselves, to others, or to property, a parent or other authorized adult caregiver should be notified.

92. What should I know about insurance and payment for treatment?

Many insurance plans provide coverage for mental health services, so be sure to call your insurance carrier to inquire about your existing benefits for mental health services. Ask about reimbursement rates for PPO plans, and check to see if any restrictions or limitations regarding the use of mental health benefits may apply. If you live in a country that provides national health care, you should inquire as to the range of treatment options offered for eating disorders recovery. If you do not have medical insurance or you earn a low income, try contacting Social Services about applying for Medicare or Medicaid. If health insurance is not available to you, you may find help from an employee assistant program, a government employee program, or a military health plan. If you are a student, try your campus health center, where services are often low in cost or free. Large universities also frequently conduct research on eating disorders and provide free treatment to

Emancipated
(when referring to a minor) A person under 18 years of age who is married or who is determined by a court of competent jurisdiction to be legally able to care for himself or herself.

Treatment and Recovery

study participants. Free support groups are available in many areas as well. The National Eating Disorders Association (NEDA) and the National Association of Anorexia Nervosa and Associated Disorders (ANAD) both provide information about free support groups located in the United States and Canada (see the Resources section for information about how to contact these organizations).

If you do not have health insurance, you should ask healthcare providers in your area about their respective out-of-pocket fees. Many therapists, community clinics, and treatment centers offer a sliding-scale fee and will attempt to negotiate a fee that you can afford. Other providers may be willing to temporarily reduce their fees or arrange a payment schedule. Some larger treatment facilities offer "scholarships" to patients in low-income situations, so be sure to investigate all of the available options. Keep in mind you cannot be denied emergency treatment for medical complications that may arise as a result of anorexia, so be sure to know where emergency medical settings are located in your immediate area.

A final note on this question: Limited access to care based on insurance benefit restrictions has historically posed a barrier to the recovery process, however a recent landmark decision by the U.S. government promises to remedy this situation. The new mental health parity law promises to end insurance discrimination by making it illegal for health insurance companies to discriminate against patients suffering from psychological or behavioral disorders. For decades, insurers have set higher co-payments and deductibles and stricter limits on treatment for addiction and mental illnesses. However, under the new law, health insurance companies will be required to provide equal coverage of mental and physical illnesses. This equivalence, or "parity," in insurance coverage will make it easier for people to obtain treatment for a wide range of conditions, including eating disorders.

The National Eating Disorders Association has put together an "Eating Disorder Survival Guide," a free and helpful resource that addresses insurance coverage issues, explains what to do if you have been denied coverage, and offers tips for fighting for appropriate care. The document is too lengthy to include here, but it can be accessed on the Internet at *www. nationaleatingdisorders.org*. If you believe your insurance company is unfairly denying coverage for eating disorders treatment, you may wish to consult an attorney who may be able to negotiate coverage or address the payment of claims. It may seem like a drastic step, but when it comes to the unfair practice of insurance companies acting as a barrier to appropriate care, you may need help receiving the intervention your family needs. In addition, you should always keep a written record to document any correspondence you have with insurance companies regarding treatment authorization.

93. What about self-help for anorexia? Can't I just try to recover on my own?

Recovery will take a great deal of self-effort, of that you can be sure. However, it is essential that you contact a professional treatment provider. Remember, anorexia is associated with a high risk for medical complications, so it is important that you be under a doctor's care. In addition, the road to recovery can be complicated and difficult at times. The additional support you will gain from a treatment team can help significantly. You may also greatly benefit from support groups and the sharing that takes place with other people who have recovered or are on the path toward healing. I really encourage you to reach out for help. You will be glad you did.

Having said this, there are some things you can do on your own to *enhance* your experience of recovery. For example, you can develop and practice certain at-home skills such as relaxation techniques and self-esteem building. I have included some helpful at-home activities, along with suggested resources for self-help that may be an effective means for supplementing and strengthening your progress toward recovery.

- Write your story. The authors of *Anorexia Nervosa: A Guide to Recovery* suggest writing the story of your life, exploring the events that were happening when you first

Keep a written record to document any correspondence you have with insurance companies.

The additional support you will gain from a treatment team can help significantly.

Treatment and Recovery

became self-conscious about your body. This exercise can take weeks or even months to complete and can help you get to know yourself better and understand how anorexia has affected you; and perhaps it will help you to cope.

- Use a self-esteem recovery workbook. *Self-Esteem: Tools for Recovery* by Lindsey Hall and Leigh Cohn and *The Self-Esteem Workbook* by Glenn R. Schiraldi are two examples.

- Keep a "feelings journal." This will help you develop greater awareness of your own feelings, thoughts, and reactions to daily events, which can in turn enhance self-awareness.

- Make a "values list" that includes things important to you, such as the activities you enjoy, the activities you would like to do more often, and the strengths that you value in people you love.

- Develop your creativity. For example, use art to develop your creative side and as a means of self-expression.

- Get connected to your spiritual side. Connect to places, people, and activities that instill hope and provide a sense of purpose and meaning outside yourself.

- Branch out to new social activities. Making new friends and interacting in new environments can reduce the isolation that comes with anorexia and provide opportunities for forming healthy and supportive relationships.

- Get connected using technology. There are more and more chat rooms, online support groups, and blogs available for those in recovery. Use resources that offer positive support for your recovery efforts. Helpful Web sites include: *www.eatingdisordersblogs.com* and *www. something-fishy.org*.

- Relax. Use relaxation techniques to assist you. Meditation, yoga, and progressive relaxation are some helpful methods. Some proven distraction techniques can also be helpful and include: deep breathing, calling a friend, taking a bath, going for a leisurely stroll, singing, drawing, painting, going to church or other place of worship, writing a letter, reciting a poem, playing a musical instrument, writing a song, and text-messaging. *The Relaxation and Stress*

Reduction Workbook, 6^(th) Edition, by Davis, Eshelman, and McKay is a popular self-help relaxation guide.

- Use a guided self-help manual *in conjunction* with psychotherapy. Several great workbooks are available that can enhance the therapy process. Suggestions can be found in the Resources section of this book.

Lynn shares:

When I started my recovery in the late 1970s there weren't the resources available that there are today. I used a 12-step program, alcoholics anonymous, as a support group even though I didn't have a drinking problem. The program did help me to stop the symptoms of the eating disorder, but much of the underlying psychology that contributed to the disorder went unresolved. As a consequence, I struggled with a lot of devastating depression while I slowly pieced together the recovery puzzle.

The process doesn't have to be so long and difficult. Recovery is hard work even with the best of resources, and the value of a good treatment team to help get you through it can't be emphasized enough. It is a tough disease to fight, and you want to give yourself every chance to beat it completely and thoroughly, and to be successful in your recovery. Anorexia most always involves denial and increasing isolation. These aspects can be next to impossible to address without outside help of some sort. A major part of recovery involves learning to consider some other perspectives, participating in honest discussions, and developing relationships with your treatment or support team, whatever that may be. Just abstaining from the symptoms of an eating disorder without addressing the underlying issues is a very difficult and unpleasant way to live. You might find other ways to cope with life that are just as bad or worse.

Sarah shares:

For a long time, I refused to believe I had a problem with my eating. Even after I was diagnosed with anorexia nervosa, I told myself that if I had gotten myself into the situation, then surely I could get myself out. I was so wrong.

Of course, there was always a certain degree of control I had over how much better I could get. I had to decide that I wanted to get better, and after that I had to work harder than I ever thought was possible to conquer my fears and let go of my anorexia. But looking back, there is no way on earth I could have made the progress I did without the help of my doctors, therapists, nutritionists, and friends at the Center for Hope of the Sierras.

I've always tended to think I'm right in any given situation. Even when I was emaciated and running myself to death, I didn't think a doctor could say or do anything to help me. But at some point in our lives, we will all find ourselves in a situation that we just can't get out of on our own. For me, anorexia was that situation, and learning to let go and let others help me was a life lesson I'm sure will continue to help me far down the road.

94. My whole life has been wrapped up in this eating disorder. How can I begin to rebuild a healthy view of myself after so long?

You touch on a very important point. For many patients, the onset of anorexia occurs during the years associated with puberty and maturation, thus delaying or interfering with the process of identity development that usually takes place during this time. The way individuals view themselves can have a significant impact on their behavior, sense-of-self, and understanding of their own personality, capabilities, and unique identity. When individuals *identify themselves with their eating disorder,* a great deal of their focus is consumed with maintaining symptoms that affect weight, shape, and appearance. A key goal of recovery, therefore, is to shift focus toward developing a more holistic, healthy, and balanced self-concept. It is important that individuals begin to understand that their true "self" is *separate from* their eating disorder. This so-called "identity-shift" takes time. Psychotherapy can help in exploring, identifying, and developing a person's own unique passions, interests, strengths, and potential, thus re-laying a new foundation for a life well lived.

It is important that individuals begin to understand that their true "self" is separate from their eating disorder.

Lynn shares:

I was greatly helped by understanding the biology of recovery. As an athlete, I believed that weight gain always came from added fat. In my recovery I added some 20 pounds to my frame. However, the weight gain was largely the result of added muscle, bone, and organ tissue. I learned the added weight, in whatever form, was necessary to help strengthen bones, as well as for starting regular periods. I focused on feeling good and feeling healthy rather than on what I weighed or how I thought I looked. I tried to change focus and get involved with new interests and activities. For example, I learned how to engineer a steam engine, which helped in developing new friends, skills, and interests. When I couldn't remember what I had for lunch that day, and didn't really care because I was so involved with running a steam engine, I knew I was on the right road to recovery. I was one of the first female steam engineers rather than a person defined by my eating disorder and how I looked or what I might weigh.

95. What are some practical things I can do to make the most of my recovery process?

That is a great question. Educating yourself about anorexia is one of the most practical and important things you can do to enhance your recovery, and you are already doing that if you are reading these words. Refer to the information contained in this book whenever you have questions or are in need of practical reminders. Also, be sure to explore the helpful resources presented in the back of this book for additional information. Next, you can practice the new skills you learn in treatment and use the recovery "tools" you acquire. The more tools you have in your recovery toolbox, the better you will be able to maintain positive change. Suggestions of practical recovery tools include:

- Be honest with your treatment team. If something is not working for you, let your team know. Share your honest thoughts, feelings, and reactions whenever possible. Your team will be able to help you most effectively when you are honest with them.

- Be active and engaged in the recovery process. Studies show that the more active, engaged, and informed a person is in the healing process, the better the prognosis for recovery.
- Ask questions. If you are unclear about a suggestion made by your team or a proposed intervention, ask for clarification. Get a second opinion if necessary. You have the right to feel confident in your treatment team.
- Talk it out. Keep in mind, miscommunication, misunderstanding, and disagreements are natural in any relationship and certainly may arise during the course of therapy. Keep the lines of communication open. No one is perfect, including your treatment team!
- Give feedback. Let your team know what is working well or what has worked well for you in the past.
- Stay in touch. If you are in outpatient therapy, you may need to find a way to stay in contact with your therapist between sessions. Discuss what will work best for you. Some therapists will respond to text messages, e-mails, or phone calls between sessions. Even as you progress in recovery, be sure to maintain a connection with your treatment team and/or schedule periodic check-ins. Think of this step as getting a recovery "booster shot."
- *Do not* ignore a potential emergency. If you feel you (or your loved one) are in crisis or are at high risk for physical complications, seek immediate help.
- Eat at regular intervals, and get plenty of rest. Maintaining a healthy weight is a key to successful recovery. Review your food plan if you notice the temptation to restrict food or to binge. If you start to lose weight, share this with your team as soon as possible.
- Try not to get back on the scale. Instead, let your doctors be the ones to weigh you, as needed. If you learn of your weight and have a strong reaction to it, be sure to address your feelings with your treatment team.
- Keep your eye on the big picture. If you do experience a setback, know that it does not mean you will be back at

square one or that you have failed in your efforts. Recovery can take a significant amount of time. Be patient with yourself and with the recovery process.

96. How can I prevent a relapse of my symptoms?

Believe it or not, asking this question is the first step toward preventing relapse! Just as education about eating disorders is an important aspect of treatment, education about relapse prevention and management is vital for staying on course during your journey of recovery. Remember that the path of recovery is not a perfect one, so bumps and turns on the road are, in fact, to be expected. Indeed, assuming that there will *not* be challenges may actually enable future roadblocks. Learning to recognize signals of potential relapse can help in knowing what to do if and when such lapses arise.

First, be aware that for hospitalized patients, attaining a normal weight prior to leaving the hospital is very important for reducing the risk of relapse. Close follow-up is the next step. The first 18 months after hospitalization carry the highest risk of relapse, so be sure to have regular checkups with your doctor, continue in psychotherapy, and receive regular input from your nutritional therapist. Next, you should know that the greatest risk for later relapse is associated with stressful life events or major life changes, even years after recovery. If you anticipate or experience a stressful situation or challenge, *prepare* instead of *panic*. Reach out to your treatment team, or, if time has elapsed and you are no longer in treatment, contact a local therapist. The same kinds of interventions you will learn in treatment are also helpful for preventing and managing relapse. Problem solving, cognitive-behavioral therapy, relaxation training, Maudsley therapy, and medication have all proven useful.

An important piece of relapse prevention is being alert to relapse warning signs so you may address any concerns early on. If you notice any of the signals from the following list,

Learning to recognize signals of potential relapse can help in knowing what to do if and when such lapses arise.

be sure to inform your treatment team; however, by the same token, do not assume the worst, as these signs can also simply be an indication that you are experiencing increased stress. In either case, addressing concerns directly will help to boost your coping skills and reduce the likelihood of experiencing a return of symptoms. So, watch for any of the following:

- Increased thoughts about weight
- Increased desire to diet, overexercise, fast, or purge
- Unexpected *or* intentional changes in weight
- Inability to sleep well
- Frequent crying, feelings of hopelessness, or other signs of depression
- Amenorrhea
- Lack of motivation
- Social isolation
- Restlessness
- Anxiety or worry
- Significant life transition or change

Lynn shares:

I have been recovered from the symptoms of anorexia and eating disorders for almost 20 years now. Periodic concerns about weight now center more on health issues. I find myself thinking I need to lose weight to maintain good cholesterol levels, joint health, or blood pressure. The years around menopause bring about some more body changes that can be triggering. I found it helpful to work with a good doctor to help balance my perspective. It is way too easy to go back to obsessive thoughts on weight and body image. I found it most helpful to concentrate on things outside of myself like relationships, family, career, and reaching out to help others. You can share your experience, strength, and hope with those who are fighting the disease. You can help in education or advocacy, or you can get involved in some other endeavor. Just maintaining that outside focus and putting yourself out there in the world goes a long way to fighting relapse. When you are not obsessing about it, your body is free to regulate your ideal weight according to its own beautiful design.

PART TEN

Prevention and Advocacy

Is anorexia preventable?

What are some examples of successful prevention programs?

What can individuals and families do to help with prevention efforts?

More . . .

97. Is anorexia preventable?

There is a growing body of evidence suggesting the effectiveness of prevention efforts. Targeting prevention efforts at those most at risk, addressing cultural support for eating disorders, and increasing **protective factors** against anorexia are all beneficial measures for prevention. Some prevention efforts come in the form of formal "programs" geared at reducing the risk of developing an eating disorder. Parents, families, former patients, and local communities also contribute immensely to prevention efforts. When we all come together, lasting change can result. It may "take a village" to raise a child well, but it takes a *culture* to combat the proliferation of eating disorders. If every one of us makes even the simplest change to combat our culture's preoccupation with thinness, it will go a long way toward eradicating these potentially deadly illnesses.

Protective factor

A characteristic that decreases a person's likelihood of developing an illness.

It takes a culture to combat the proliferation of eating disorders.

98. What are some examples of successful prevention programs?

Research shows that the most effective efforts at prevention are those that try to reach kids early, include parents, and encourage community involvement. Additionally, interactive and participatory prevention efforts are best, whenever possible. In fact, some studies suggest that strictly didactic presentations may even be counterproductive, especially for those in high-risk populations. It is also important for prevention efforts to support the development of protective factors that may reduce the risk of developing anorexia. Studies show that protective factors include high self-esteem, high **self-efficacy**, optimism, creativity, spirituality, a supportive family network, positive role models, participation in extracurricular activities, problem-solving skills, and the participation in non-elite sports.

Self-efficacy

The impression or judgment of one's own capabilities.

Prevention strategies vary depending on the target audience and scope of the program. Studies show that school-based prevention programs can be helpful, particularly when teachers, coaches, and other staff are educated about prevention prior to intervening with students. Making changes to the social environments of high-risk populations is a key factor to the success of prevention efforts. For example, one pilot study in 1999 worked toward environmental changes at an elite ballet school. Peer behavior, staff behavior, curriculum, and school policies were just some of the areas in which sweeping changes occurred. These changes resulted in a reduction of eating disorder symptoms among students. Other programs such as Athletes Targeting Healthy Exercise and Nutrition Alternatives (ATHENA) have shown promise in research studies. ATHENA promotes exercise and nutrition as alternatives to reliance on diet supplements or unhealthy approaches to conditioning and weight control. ATHENA was one of two prevention programs to receive an award for its efforts from *Sports Illustrated.*

Programs that teach media literacy have become increasingly popular in recent years and have produced promising results. These efforts encourage critical viewing of media images to reduce the impact of unhealthy messages pertaining to weight and body image. Researchers have emphasized the "Five A's" of effective media literacy programs: Awareness of media use, Analysis of media content, Activism (e.g., letters of praise or protest sent to advertisers), Advocacy for healthy alternative media messages, and increased understanding of who has Access to mass media in order to participate in media in positive ways (Levine and Smolak 2006). The National Eating Disorders Association (NEDA) has produced a media literacy curriculum for middle and high school girls entitled "Go Girls!" The program helps girls to recognize and analyze body image messages from the media, to strengthen their self-confidence, and to voice their own opinions. NEDA has also produced a curriculum for children in grades 4–6 entitled *Healthy Body Image: Teaching Kids to Eat and Love Their Bodies Too!* (2nd Edition), authored by clinical social worker Kathy J. Kater. Similar dual-gender curriculums have been developed by other eating disorders organizations. A list of available curriculums can be obtained from Gürze Books LLC Publishing Company (*www.bulimia.com*).

Prevention and Advocacy

In addition, general health promotion programs have proven to be a good way to reduce the risk of eating disorders. A 1999 issue of *European Eating Disorders Review* identified practical goals for health promotion strategies aimed at increasing self-efficacy and reducing the risk of illness. These goals include promoting healthy stress management, increasing self-esteem, increasing confidence in expressing one's needs and emotions, reducing perfectionism, enforcing healthier eating habits, and connecting self-esteem to factors other than weight and appearance.

While prevention efforts should start early, studies do show that prevention programs geared toward adults can be successful as well. Discussion groups that focus on positive body image, address the negative effects of dieting, and promote media literacy training are just three of the many approaches to adult prevention that have yielded positive results. Toward that end, NEDA recently launched a "media watchdog" program created to improve media messages about size, weight, and beauty. The program brings students, educators, health professionals, parents, eating disorders sufferers, and concerned consumers together to encourage companies and advertisers to send healthy media messages about body shape and size. Participants are trained to recognize and celebrate advertisements that send healthy body image messages and are encouraged to take the time to express concerns about advertisements that send negative body image messages. To date, over 1000 volunteer media watchdogs have joined this effort.

One of the largest prevention campaigns that NEDA has undertaken is their annual Eating Disorders Awareness Week (NEDAW). The organization sets aside the last week of February each year to promote awareness, treatment, and prevention of eating disorders. NEDAW has become a national movement, and local healthcare professionals, organizations, and individuals are encouraged to host NEDAW events in their respective communities. To learn more about NEDAW or about becoming a "media watchdog," visit NEDA's Web site at *www.nationaleatingdisorders.org*.

99. *What can individuals and families do to help with prevention efforts?*

You would be surprised at how far reaching individual prevention efforts can be! When teachers, coaches, parents, camp counselors, former patients, and others each do their part to change the way people think about anorexia and eating disorders, the ripple effect can be tremendous! Whether it is sending a letter to the editor of a fashion magazine, joining fundraising efforts for eating disorders organizations, consciousness-raising by a teacher in the classroom, or simply raising a child to appreciate the diversity of body types, much can be accomplished when we join toward the common cause of eradicating anorexia in our day. Perhaps reading this book has inspired your own ideas for becoming involved in prevention and **advocacy** efforts. Here are some suggestions of ways you can assist prevention efforts on an individual level:

- Discourage your loved ones from restrictive forms of dieting. Emphasize health and fitness as a goal instead of slenderness.
- Teach your family to think critically about unhealthy messages pertaining to body shape and physical appearance.
- Get the word out about the seriousness of anorexia and other eating disorders. Share eating disorders resources with teachers, coaches, and local PTA.
- Keep a scrapbook of positive body images by cutting out ads from magazines.
- Do not subscribe to magazines that promote a distorted thin ideal or objectify women. Instead, try to support media that promotes a healthy body image.
- Model a healthy attitude about weight, shape, food, and exercise in your own home. Eat together as a family whenever you can. Promote a "health at any size" mentality in your social circles.
- Do not criticize anyone's appearance or eating habits, and do not tease about weight or shape. If you hear others do so, ask them to stop. Do not allow teasing

Much can be accomplished when we join toward the common cause of eradicating anorexia in our day.

Advocacy
Active support of a cause, speaking out about a concern, or representing the cause or interest of another.

Prevention and Advocacy

about weight in your classrooms, on your playgrounds, or in your home. If your child makes disparaging comments about his or her *own* appearance, sit down and have a conversation about how he or she is feeling.

- Love your children unconditionally. Compliment your children for who they are, not how they look. Give equal opportunities and encouragement to sons and daughters. Do not encourage perfectionism; encourage assertiveness and the healthy expression of feelings.

- Teach media literacy in your own home. If your child appears to idolize a thin celebrity, consider this an opportunity to have a conversation about body image and attractiveness. Connect your growing boys and girls to healthy role models.

- Make a list of companies that consistently use images of a thin ideal in their advertising, and send a letter to their marketing departments. Share how their ad affected you. Let them know you will be more likely to buy their products if they advertise in a way that challenges society's thin ideal.

- Volunteer with an organization that helps to combat eating disorders. Consider making a financial donation for their continued efforts.

- If you are a patient, consider participating in a research study. Participants are needed on an ongoing basis, and you may be able to receive free treatment in return for your participation. A list of ongoing research studies can be found on a number of reputable Internet sites (see the Resources section for a list).

- If you think someone you love may have an eating disorder, speak to him or her about getting help.

100. What is eating disorders advocacy, and how do I become involved?

Eating disorders advocacy involves speaking out about the seriousness of these illnesses and becoming active in efforts aimed at bringing about change in research funding, treatment access, and community education. There are many ways to become involved in advocacy efforts. You can be involved in an informal way, such as by sharing in your neighborhood the importance of research and treatment for eating disorders, or by supporting a local or national eating disorders organization. You can also choose a more formal means for involvement, such as meeting with your local legislators and advocating policy changes that will positively affect the battle against these devastating illnesses.

Advocacy efforts really do make a difference. Take for example legislation passed in the summer of 2007 by the New York State Senate. Legislators in that state established the Child Performer Advisory Board to Prevent Eating Disorders. This Board will be developing guidelines for the employment of child models along with educational programs aimed at preventing and treating eating disorders. More recently, in April of 2008, the first comprehensive eating disorder legislation in U.S. history was introduced in Washington, DC. A project of the Eating Disorders Coalition, a Washington, DC-based U.S. advocacy organization, and in cooperation with Representatives Patrick Kennedy (D-RI) and Michael Ferguson (R-NJ), the FREED Act (The Federal Response to Eliminate Eating Disorders) is important legislation for supporting eating disorders research, treatment, prevention, and education. And in October of 2008, the U.S. Government passed a new law that requires health insurance companies nationwide to provide coverage for mental health treatment on an equal basis with medical care, a concept known as mental health parity. Legislation such as this comes about with the help of ordinary citizens and organizations who commit to being a voice for change. You can join that chorus of voices through your own participation, however great or small. With this aim in mind, you will find a list of organizations that are actively involved in eating disorders advocacy in the Resources section that follows.

Prevention and Advocacy

Internationally, 2008 witnessed the launching of a global initiative sponsored by the Academy for Eating Disorders (AED). The "Worldwide Charter for Action on Eating Disorders" attempts to define rights and expectations for patients and their families with regard to health policies and practices worldwide. The goal is to form a united coalition that can persuade policy makers around the globe to commit to supporting effective, affordable, and quality treatment for eating disorders. You can learn more about the Charter by visiting the AED Web site at *www.aedweb.org*.

Advocacy with the media has also yielded many positive outcomes. Even large corporations have become a part of the advocacy process. For example, in 2004, Dove launched the Campaign for Real Beauty, featuring real women—not models—in advertisements for Dove products. This is an attempt to promote natural beauty, feature a variety of body images, and combat the thin ideal. Globally, we are witnessing media advocacy as it becomes a worldwide effort. For example, in March of 2008, Italian authorities mounted a $1.5 million anti-anorexia campaign geared toward combating the illness. In September of 2008, members of the European Parliament adopted an initiative report on advertising, noting that "portrayals of the ideal body image can adversely affect the self-esteem of women and men, particularly teenagers and those susceptible to eating disorders." The parliament called on advertisers to "consider more carefully their use of extremely thin women to advertise products." (see Question 25 for other international advocacy developments). It is encouraging to witness such helpful efforts in regions that are known for fashion and image consciousness.

When we each become active in anorexia advocacy efforts, we contribute to increasing understanding, improving access to care, and enhancing the quality and effectiveness of treatments for the illness. Together, let us unite toward the goal of making anorexia nervosa a thing of the past.

Appendix A

The Eating Attitudes Test (EAT-26)

The EAT-26 may help you determine if you need to speak to a mental health professional or a physician about getting help for an eating disorder. Completing the EAT-26 will take you about 2 minutes.

The EAT-26 is the most widely used screening measure for helping individuals determine if they have an eating disorder that needs professional attention. The EAT-26 is a measure of symptoms and concerns that are characteristic of eating disorders. In 1982, the test was updated and shortened to the current 26-item version, known as the EAT-26. The EAT-26 is designed to be either self-administered or administered by health professionals, school counselors, coaches, camp counselors, and others. The EAT-26 is not designed to make a diagnosis of an eating disorder or to take the place of a professional diagnosis or consultation.

The EAT-26 alone does not diagnose an eating disorder. In fact, no test or screening instrument has been shown to be highly efficient as the sole means of identifying an eating disorder. Only a qualified healthcare professional can provide a diagnosis. However, the EAT-26 can be a first step in the screening process, with the second step being a consultation and evaluation with a qualified professional. Early screening is important because an eating disorder identified in its early stages can lead a person to seek earlier treatment, thereby reducing the risk of serious physical and psychological complications. The EAT-26 can be a particularly useful tool for assessing "eating disorder risk."

All self-report measures require open and honest responses in order to provide accurate information. The fact that most people provide honest responses means the EAT-26 usually provides very useful information about the eating symptoms and concerns that are common in eating disorders.

Height _____
Current weight _____
Highest weight (excluding pregnancy) _____
Lowest adult weight _____

Do you participate in athletics at any of the following levels?

☐ Intramural
☐ Inter-collegiate
☐ Recreational
☐ High school teams

Please check a response for each of the following statements:

	Always	Usually	Often	Sometimes	Rarely	Never	Score
1. I am terrified about being overweight.	☐	☐	☐	☐	☐	☐	___
2. I avoid eating when I am hungry.	☐	☐	☐	☐	☐	☐	___
3. I find myself preoccupied with food.	☐	☐	☐	☐	☐	☐	___
4. I have gone on eating binges where I feel that I may not be able to stop.	☐	☐	☐	☐	☐	☐	___
5. I cut my food into small pieces.	☐	☐	☐	☐	☐	☐	___
6. I am aware of the calorie content of foods that I eat.	☐	☐	☐	☐	☐	☐	___
7. I particularly avoid food with high carbohydrate content (e.g., bread, rice, potatoes, etc.).	☐	☐	☐	☐	☐	☐	___
8. I feel that others would prefer if I ate more.	☐	☐	☐	☐	☐	☐	___
9. I vomit after I have eaten.	☐	☐	☐	☐	☐	☐	___
10. I feel extremely guilty after eating.	☐	☐	☐	☐	☐	☐	___
11. I am preoccupied with a desire to be thinner.	☐	☐	☐	☐	☐	☐	___
12. I think about burning up calories when I exercise.	☐	☐	☐	☐	☐	☐	___

	Always	Usually	Often	Sometimes	Rarely	Never	Score
13. Other people think that I am too thin.	☐	☐	☐	☐	☐	☐	___
14. I am preoccupied with the thought of having fat on my body.	☐	☐	☐	☐	☐	☐	___
15. I take longer than others to eat my meals.	☐	☐	☐	☐	☐	☐	___
16. I avoid foods with sugar in them.	☐	☐	☐	☐	☐	☐	___
17. I eat diet foods.	☐	☐	☐	☐	☐	☐	___
18. I feel that food controls my life.	☐	☐	☐	☐	☐	☐	___
19. I display self-control around food.	☐	☐	☐	☐	☐	☐	___
20. I feel that others pressure me to eat.	☐	☐	☐	☐	☐	☐	___
21. I give too much time and thought to food.	☐	☐	☐	☐	☐	☐	___
22. I feel uncomfortable after eating sweets.	☐	☐	☐	☐	☐	☐	___
23. I engage in dieting behavior.	☐	☐	☐	☐	☐	☐	___
24. I like my stomach to be empty.	☐	☐	☐	☐	☐	☐	___
25. I have the impulse to vomit after meals.	☐	☐	☐	☐	☐	☐	___
26. I enjoy trying new rich foods.	☐	☐	☐	☐	☐	☐	___

Total Score (see below for scoring instructions) _____

Scoring The Eating Attitudes Test

For all items **except #26**, each of the responses receives the following value:

Always = 3
Usually = 2
Often = 1
Sometimes = 0
Rarely = 0
Never = 0

Appendix A

For #26;

> Always = 0
> Usually = 0
> Often = 0
> Sometimes = 1
> Rarely = 2
> Never = 3

Interpreting high scores (20 or higher)—If people have EAT-26 scores of 20 or higher, it does not necessarily indicate they have an eating disorder, but it does indicate concerns regarding body weight, body shape, and eating. If you have a score of 20 or higher, please seek the advice of a qualified mental health professional who has experience with treating eating disorders. The only way to determine if you meet the diagnostic criteria for an eating disorder is through an interview and follow-up evaluation with a qualified professional, such as your personal physician or an eating disorder treatment specialist.

Interpreting low scores (below 20)—Self-report measures require open and honest responses for accuracy, so denial can create a problem for interpreting test scores. Therefore, a person who has EAT-26 scores below 20 can still have clinically significant eating disorder symptoms or a formal eating disorder. Collateral information from parents, teammates, and coaches can correct for denial, limited self-disclosure, and answering in a socially "acceptable" way.

Other important pieces of information about weight-control behaviors—Have any of the following weight-control behaviors been present in the previous 6 months?

- Self-reported binge eating
- Self-induced vomiting
- Laxative use
- Eating disorder treatment

Contact a healthcare professional if you feel you are in need of assistance. If you believe you are in crisis or in need of immediate attention, call 911, or visit your local emergency room.

SOURCE: Garner, D. M., Olmsted, M. P., Bohr, Y., and Garfinkel, P. E. (1982). The eating attitudes test: Psychometric features and clinical correlates. *Psychological Medicine 12*: 871–878. (This questionnaire is made available by permission of the authors.)

Appendix B

Resources

Resources for Treatment Referrals, Information, and Family Support

Academy for Eating Disorders (AED)
111 Deer Lake Road, Suite 100
Deerfield, IL 60015
Phone: (847) 498-4274
www.aedweb.org

American Dietetic Association (nutrition information and dietitian referrals)
120 South Riverside Plaza, Suite 2000
Chicago, IL 60606-6995
Phone: (800) 877-1600
www.eatright.org

American Psychological Association
750 First Street N.E.
Washington, DC 20002-4242
Phone: (800) 374-2721
www.apa.org

beat (Beating Eating Disorders) (in the United Kingdom)
103 Prince of Wales Road
Norwich NR1 1DW; United Kingdom
Phone: 0870-770-3256
www.b-eat.co.uk/Home

Eating Disorders Referral and Information Center
Phone: (800) 843-7274
www.edreferral.com

Gürze Books Eating Disorders Resources (free articles about anorexia, treatment referrals, and free catalogue of resources)
5145 B Avenida Encinas
Carlsbad, CA 92008
Phone: (800) 756-7533
www.bulimia.com

International Association of Eating Disorder Professionals (IAEDP)
PO Box 1295
Pekin, IL 61555-1295
Phone: (800) 800-8126
www.iaedp.com

Multiservice Eating Disorders Association (MEDA)
92 Pearl Street
Newton, MA 02458
Phone: (866) 343-MEDA
www.medainc.org

National Alliance on Mental Illness (NAMI)
Colonial Place Three
2107 Wilson Boulevard, Suite 300
Arlington, VA 22201-3042
Phone: (800) 950-6264
www.nami.org

National Association of Anorexia Nervosa and Associated Disorders (ANAD)
PO Box 7
Highland Park, IL 60035
Phone: (847) 831-3438
www.anad.org

National Centre for Eating Disorders (in the United Kingdom)
54 New Road
Esher, Surrey KT10 9NU; United Kingdom
Phone: 0845-838-2040
www.eating-disorders.org.uk

National Eating Disorder Information Centre (in Canada)
ES 7-421, 200 Elizabeth Street
Toronto, Ontario M5G 2C4
Phone: (866) 633-4230 (toll free in Canada) or (416) 340-4156
www.nedic.ca

National Eating Disorders Association (NEDA)
603 Stewart Street, Suite 803
Seattle, WA 98101
Phone: (800) 931-2237
www.nationaleatingdisorders.org

Something Fishy
Phone: (866) 690-7239
www.something-fishy.org

Other Helpful General Information-Based Web sites

Anorexia Nervosa and Related Eating Disorders, Inc. (ANRED)
www.anred.com

Mirror-Mirror (general eating disorders information)
www.mirror-mirror.org

Sari Shepphird, Ph.D. (links to free articles and other resources for patients, families, and professionals)
www.drshepp.com

Sports, Cardiovascular, and Wellness Nutritionists (dietitian and nutritionist referral Web site)
www.scandpg.org

USDA Nutrition Information
www.nutrition.gov

Body Image Resources
Web sites

Body Positive
www.bodypositive.com

Body Image Health Resources (prevention curriculum by Kathy Kater, LICSW)
www.BodyImageHealth.org

The BodySense Program (based in Canada)
www.bodysense.ca

Books

Maine, M., and Kelly, J. (2005). *The body myth: Adult women and the pressure to be perfect.* New Jersey: John Wiley & Sons, Inc.

Richardson, B. L., and Rehr, E. (2001). *101 ways to help your daughter love her body.* New York: (Quill) HarperCollins Publishers.

Eating Disorders Advocacy Organizations

Academy for Eating Disorders (AED)
111 Deer Lake Road, Suite 100
Deerfield, IL 60015
Phone: (847) 498-4274
www.aedweb.org

Eating Disorders Coalition for Research, Policy, and Action (EDC)
720 7th Street NW, Suite 300
Washington, DC 20001-3902
Phone: (202) 543-9570
www.eatingdisorderscoalition.org

National Association of Anorexia Nervosa and Associated Disorders (ANAD)
PO Box 7
Highland Park, IL 60035
Phone: (847) 831-3438
www.anad.org

National Eating Disorders Association (NEDA)
603 Stewart Street, Suite 803
Seattle, WA 98101
Phone: (800) 931-2237
www.nationaleatingdisorders.org

Maudsley Therapy Resources
Web sites

www.eatingwithyouranorexic.com

www.MaudsleyParents.org

Books

Herrin, M., and Matsumoto, N. (2007). *The parent's guide to eating disorders: Supporting self-esteem, healthy eating, and positive body image*, 2nd ed. Carlsbad, CA: Gürze Books.

Lock, J., and le Grange, D. (2005). *Help your teenager beat an eating disorder.* New York: The Guilford Press.

Treasure, J., Smith, G., and Crane, A. (2007). *Skills-based learning for caring for a loved one with an eating disorder: The new Maudsley method.* New York: Routledge.

Treatment

University of California, San Diego Intensive Family Treatment Eating Disorders Program

http://eatingdisorders.ucsd.edu/IFT.html

Media Education and Awareness
Web sites

About-Face

www.about-face.org

Jean Kilbourne (media awareness resource Web site)

www.jeankilbourne.com

Just Think

www.justthink.org

Books

Brashich, A. D. (2006). *All made up: A girl's guide to seeing through celebrity hype and celebrating real beauty.* New York: (Walker Books for Young Readers) Walker and Company.

Graydon, S. (2003). *Made you look: How advertising works and why you should know.* New York: Annick Press.

Kilbourne, J. (2000). *Can't buy me love: How advertising changes the way we think and feel.* New York: (Free Press) Simon & Schuster, Inc.

Videos

Kilbourne, J. (2000). *Killing us softly 3: Advertising's image of women* [DVD]. Northampton, MA: Media Education Foundation.

Lazarus, M., (Producer/Director) and Wunderlich, R. (Producer/Director). (2000). *The strength to resist: Media's impact on women and girls* [DVD]. Cambridge, MA: Cambridge Documentary Films.

Research Study Listings

www.anad.org

www.anred.com

www.bodypositive.com

www.bulimia.com

www.edreferral.com

www.something-fishy.org

Workbooks and Self-Help Resources

Claiborn, J., and Pedrick, C. (2002). *The BDD workbook: Overcome body dysmorphic disorder and end body image obsessions*. Oakland, CA: New Harbinger Publications, Inc.

Davis, M., Eshelman, E. R., and McKay, M. (2008). *The relaxation and stress reduction workbook*, 6th ed. Oakland, CA: New Harbinger Publications, Inc.

Dellasega, C. (2005). *The starving family companion workbook: A workbook for parents caring for children with eating disorders*. Fredonia, Wisconsin: Champion Press.

Eivors, A., and Nesbitt, S. (2005). *Hunger for understanding: A workbook for helping young people to understand and overcome anorexia nervosa*. West Sussex, England: John Wiley & Sons, Inc.

Goodman, L. J., and Villapiano, M. (2001). *Eating disorders: The journey to recovery workbook*. New York: (Brunner-Routledge) Taylor & Francis.

Hall, L., and Cohn, L. (1990). *Self-esteem: Tools for recovery*. Carlsbad, CA: Gürze Books.

Kano, S. (1989). *Making peace with food: Freeing yourself from the diet/weight obsession*. New York: Harper & Row.

Koenig, K. R. (2007). *The food and feelings workbook: A full course meal on emotional health*. Carlsbad, CA: Gürze Books.

Schiraldi, G.R. (2001). *The self-esteem workbook*. Oakland, CA: New Harbinger Publications, Inc.

Walsh, B. T., and Cameron, V. L. (2005). *If your adolescent has an eating disorder: An essential resource for parents*. New York: Oxford University Press.

Other Recommended Books

Anderson, A. E., Cohn, L., and Holbrook, T. (2000). *Making weight: Men's conflicts with food, weight, shape, and appearance.* Carlsbad, CA: Gürze Books.

Brumberg, J. J. (2000). *Fasting girls: The history of anorexia nervosa.* New York: Vintage Books (Random House).

Hall, L., and Ostroff, M. (1998). *Anorexia nervosa: A guide to recovery.* Carlsbad, CA: Gürze Books.

Heaton, J.A., and Strauss, C. J. (2005). *Talking to eating disorders: Simple ways to support someone with anorexia, bulimia, binge eating, or body image issues.* New York: New American Library (Penguin).

Institute for Research and Education Health System. (1999). *How did this happen? A practical guide to understanding eating disorders for teachers, parents, and coaches.* Minnesota: Author.

Katzman, D. K., and Pinhas, L. (2005). *Help for eating disorders: A parent's guide to symptoms, causes and treatments.* Toronto, Ontario: Robert Rose, Inc.

Koenig, K.R. (2005). *The rules of "normal eating": A commonsense approach for dieters, overeaters, undereaters, emotional eaters, and everyone in between!* Carlsbad, CA: Gürze Books.

Kolodny, N. J. (2004). *The beginner's guide to eating disorders recovery.* Carlsbad, CA: Gürze Books.

Liu, A. (2008). *Gaining: The truth about life after eating disorders.* New York: (Hachette Book Groups) Warner Books.

Siegel, M., Brisman, J., and Weinshel, M. (2009). *Surviving an eating disorder, Third edition: Strategies for family and friends.* New York: (Collins Living) HarperCollins Publisher Inc.

Smeltzer, D., with Smeltzer, A. L. (2006). *Andrea's voice: Silenced by bulimia: Her story and her mother's journey through grief toward understanding.* Carlsbad, CA: Gürze Books.

Strober, M., and Schneider, M. (2006). *Just a little too thin: How to pull your child back from the brink of an eating disorder.* Cambridge, MA: De Capo Press.

Winfree, W. (Ed.) (2007). *We are more than beautiful: 46 real teen girls speak out about beauty, happiness, love and life.* Naperville, IL: Sourcebooks, Inc.

Appendix B

Bibliography

Bruch, H. (1978). *The golden cage: The enigma of anorexia nervosa.* Cambridge, MA: Harvard University Press.

Cooper, Z., and Fairburn, C. G. (1987). The Eating Disorder Examination: A semi-structured interview for the assessment of the specific psychopathology of eating disorders. *International Journal of Eating Disorders* 6: 1–8.

Fairburn, C. G., and Beglin, S. J. (1994). Assessment of eating disorders: Interview or self-report. *International Journal of Eating Disorders* 16: 363–370.

Fairburn, C. G., Cooper, Z., Doll, H. A., and Welch, S. L. (1999). Risk factors for anorexia nervosa: Three integrated case-control comparisons. *Archives of General Psychiatry* 56: 468–476.

Garner, D. M. (1997). Psychoeducational principles in treatment. In D. M. Garner and P. E. Garfinkel (Eds.) *Handbook of treatment for eating disorders,* 2nd ed (pp. 145–177). New York: The Guilford Press.

Garner, D. M., and Olmstead, M. P. (1984). *Eating disorder inventory manual.* Psychological Assessment Resources, Inc.

Gordon, R. A. (2000). *Eating disorders: Anatomy of a social epidemic.* Malden, MA: Blackwell Publishers.

Hall, L., and Ostroff, M. (1999). *Anorexia nervosa: A guide to recovery.* Carlsbad, CA: Gürze Books.

Hausenblas, H. A., and Symons Downs, D. (2002). How much is too much? The development and validation of the Exercise Dependence Scale. *Psychology & Health* 17: 387–404.

Herzog, D. B., and Eddy, K. T. (2007). Diagnosis, epidemiology, and clinical course of eating disorders. In J. Yager and P. S. Powers (Eds.) *Clinical manual of eating disorders* (pp.1–29). Washington, DC: American Psychiatric Publishing, Inc.

Hsu, L. K. (1988). The outcome of anorexia nervosa: A reappraisal. *Psychological Medicine* 18: 807–812.

Jacobs, B., and Isaacs, S. (1986). Pre-puberty anorexia nervosa: A retrospective controlled study. *Journal of Child Psychology and Psychiatry* 27: 237–250.

Kano, S. (1989). *Making peace with food: Freeing yourself from the diet/weight obsession.* New York: Harper & Row.

Kilbourne, J. (2000). *Can't buy me love: How advertising changes the way we think and feel.* New York: (Free Press) Simon & Schuster, Inc.

Kolodny, N. J. (2004). *The beginner's guide to eating disorders recovery.* Carlsbad, CA: Gürze Books.

Levine, M.P., and Smolak, L. (1998). The mass media and disordered eating: Implications for primary prevention. In W. Vandereycken and G. Noordenbos (Eds.) *The Prevention of Eating Disorders* (pp. 23–56). London: The Athlone Press.

Levine, M.P., and Smolak, L. (2005). *The prevention of eating problems and eating disorders: Theory, research, and practice.* Mahwah, New Jersey: Lawrence Erlbaum Associates, Inc., Publishers.

Lock, J., and le Grange, D. (2005). *Help your teenager beat an eating disorder.* New York: The Guilford Press.

Mickley, D. (2004). Medication for anorexia nervosa and bulimia nervosa. *Eating Disorders Today* 2(4): 1 and 15.

Olson, K. (2003). *Killing us softly: 3 handouts* [Electronic Version]. Northampton, MA: Media Education Foundation.

Satter, E. (1999). *Secrets of feeding a healthy family.* Madison, WI: Kelcy Press.

Shepphird, S. (2007). Dangerous inspiration: A subculture that supports anorexia nervosa. *The Los Angeles Psychologist* 3: 12–13.

Silverman, J. A. (1997). Anorexia nervosa: Historical perspective on treatment. In D. M. Garner and P. E. Garfinkel (Eds.) *Handbook of treatment for eating disorders,* 2nd ed. (pp. 3–10). New York: The Guilford Press.

Smeltzer, D., and Smeltzer, A. L. (2006). *Andrea's voice: Silenced by bulimia: Her story and her mother's journey through grief toward understanding.* Carlsbad, CA: Gürze Books.

Vandereycken, W., and Van Deth, R. (2001). *From fasting saints to anorexic girls: The history of self-starvation.* London: The Continuum International Publishing Group.

Villapiano, M., and Goodman, L. J. (2001). *Eating disorders: Time for change.* Philadelphia, PA: (Brunner-Routledge) Taylor & Francis.

Walsh, B. T., and Cameron, V. L. (2005). *If your adolescent has an eating disorder: An essential resource for parents.* New York: Oxford University Press.

Wonderlich, S. A. (2002). Personality and eating disorders. In C. G. Fairburn and K. D. Brownell (Eds.) *Eating disorders and obesity: A comprehensive handbook,* 2nd ed. (pp. 204–209). New York: The Guilford Press.

Zerbe, K. J. (2007). Psychodynamic management of eating disorders. In J. Yager and P. S. Powers (Eds.) *Clinical manual of eating disorders.* (pp. 307–334). Washington, DC: American Psychiatric Publishing, Inc.

Glossary

A

Acculturation: Adapting to another culture or modification of one's culture through contact with another culture.

Addison's disease: A disease caused by a deficiency of hormones that are produced by the adrenal gland. Symptoms may include weight loss, fatigue, and vomiting.

Advocacy: Active support of a cause, speaking out about a concern, or representing the cause or interest of another.

Aftercare: Care services offered to a patient after he or she is discharged from a hospital or treatment program.

Aggregate death rate: Sum or total death rate over time.

Alexithymia: A trait characterized by the inability to identify and describe emotions, confusion about one's own feelings, and/or an apparent lack of consideration about one's own personal experiences.

Amenorrhea: The absence of menstrual periods in females.

Amphetamines: A class of drugs that has a stimulant effect on the central nervous system of the body.

Androgens: Male sex hormones, responsible for the development of male secondary sex characteristics.

Antecedent: Preceding event or cause.

Anxiety: A state of worry, fear, apprehension, uneasiness, or distress. Physical symptoms such as dizziness, lightheadedness, or shortness of breath may or may not also occur.

APGAR: A test to determine the physical health of a newborn baby. The total score is based on five categories: color, cry, muscle tone, respiration, and reflexes.

Arrhythmia: An abnormal or irregular rhythm of the heart.

Attention deficit hyperactivity disorder (ADHD): A persistent pattern of inattention and hyperactivity or impulsivity. The inattention may be present in academic, work, or social situations. Feelings of restlessness are common.

Avoidant personality disorder (AVPD): A persistent pattern of social inhibition, feelings of inadequacy, and extreme sensitivity to the opinions of others.

B

Binge-eating: Eating a significantly large amount of food during a given period of time.

Blood urea nitrogen: A blood test that helps to assess kidney function by measuring a waste product excreted by the kidneys.

Body dysmorphic disorder (BDD): A severe form of body image disturbance characterized by an excessive concern or preoccupation with a perceived defect in one's appearance.

Body mass index (BMI): A measurement used by physicians and other eating disorders professionals as an indicator of total body fat.

Bone density test: A test that measures the strength and density of bones; often used to determine the risk of developing osteoporosis. Also called bone mineral density (BMD) test.

Bulimia nervosa: An eating disorder characterized by recurrent episodes of binge eating followed by inappropriate compensatory behavior, such as vomiting; misuse of laxatives, diuretics, enemas, or other medications; and/or fasting or excessive exercise. There are two subtypes of bulimia nervosa: purging type and non-purging type.

C

Colitis: An inflammation of the large intestine (colon). Symptoms may include abdominal pain, fever, and severe diarrhea.

Comorbidity: The occurrence of more than one illness, disease, or diagnosable condition at the same time.

Creatinine: A waste substance produced by the muscles. Measuring the creatinine level in the blood gives an indication of kidney functioning.

D

Delayed gastric emptying: A decreased rate of emptying of the content in the stomach; also called gastroparesis. Delayed gastric emptying can cause nausea, vomiting, feeling full after a small meal, bloating, abdominal pain, and heartburn.

Delirium: An acute state of mental confusion with a sudden onset, usually reversible; includes impaired concentration, disorientation, anxiety, and sometimes hallucinations.

Dependent personality disorder: A pattern of persistent and excessive psychological dependence on others, coupled with fears of separation, beginning by early adulthood and present in a variety of contexts.

Depression: A significant disturbance in mood characterized by such symptoms as tearfulness, social withdrawal, irritability, lack of pleasure, sleeping and eating changes, and low energy levels.

Diabetes mellitus: A condition or disease in which the body is unable to appropriately control blood-sugar (glucose) levels. The two types of diabetes are referred to as insulin-dependent (Type I) and non-insulin dependent (Type II).

Diagnostic interview: A structured or semi-structured interview of a patient, conducted by a healthcare professional in order to establish an accurate diagnosis of illness or condition.

Didactic: Intending to instruct or educate.

Dopamine: A brain chemical, or neurotransmitter, which has been associated with the areas of the brain that regulate movement, mood, emotion, motivation, and pleasure.

DSM-IV-TR: Abbreviated title of the *Diagnostic and Statistical Manual of Mental Disorders, Fourth Edition, Text Revision;* a manual that qualified mental health professionals use to diagnose mental illnesses.

E

Eating disorder: A severe disturbance in eating behaviors that results in an altered consumption of food and may significantly impair physical or mental health. An eating disorder is not diagnosed when the disturbed eating behaviors are the direct result of a general medical condition.

Edema: An accumulation of excess fluid in the tissues of the body.

EDNOS: Abbreviation for "eating disorder, not otherwise specified"; a diagnostic classification for several varieties of eating disorder symptoms classified in the *DSM-IV-TR.*

Efficacy: The extent to which an intervention produces an effect or beneficial result.

Electrolytes: Salts that are found in the body, the most common of which are sodium, potassium, and chloride. A healthy balance of electrolytes is needed to maintain normal body function.

Emancipated: (when referring to a minor) A person under 18 years of age who is married or who is determined by a court of competent jurisdiction to be legally able to care for himself or herself.

Emetic: An agent that induces vomiting.

Enteral: A method of substance delivery where nutrients are given directly into the gastrointestinal tract.

Epidemiologist: A person who studies the presence of disease in a population.

Estrogen: Female hormone produced by the ovaries. It stimulates the development of secondary sexual characteristics and induces menstruation in women.

Etiology: The cause or origin of a disease, condition, or illness.

Evidence-based treatment: Treatment that seeks to apply the results of research evidence in establishing specific clinical guidelines for treatment effectiveness.

Externally oriented thinking: Thinking that tends to focus on external events rather than inner emotional experiences.

F

Food exchange system (or food exchange program): A dietary approach

Glossary

or special meal plan in which foods are categorized by food group (e.g., starches, vegetables) and serving size.

Functional magnetic resonance imaging (fMRI): A type of brain scan used to study activity in the brain. An fMRI shows which structures are active during particular mental operations.

G

Gastroparesis: Nerve or muscle damage in the stomach that causes slow digestion and gastric emptying, vomiting, nausea, or bloating.

Genetic predisposition: An inherited genetic pattern that may make a person more susceptible to a disease or condition.

Ghrelin: A hormone that relays messages between the digestive system and the brain to stimulate appetite.

Glucose: A type of sugar found in the blood and a source of energy for the body.

Gonadotropin: A group of hormones that affect the growth and function of the sex glands.

H

Hereditability factor: A calculation of the contribution made by genes to the causation of a disorder or disease.

Hypnotherapy: The use of hypnosis in therapy. In hypnotherapy, a patient is guided to a state of focused relaxation to facilitate behavioral, emotional, or attitudinal change.

I

Incidence: The number of new cases of a disease in a defined population within a specified period of time.

Individuation: The developmental process of forming one's individual personality.

Insulin: A hormone produced by the pancreas that helps the body regulate blood-sugar level.

Interoceptive cues: Sensitivity to sensations that occur inside the body (e.g., gastrointestinal sensations, cardiac sensations).

Intravenously: Injection of a substance or medication into a vein.

L

Lanugo: A fine, downy white hair that may grow on the body as a result of malnutrition.

Leptin: A protein hormone that helps the body regulate appetite and the metabolism of fats.

M

Meal plan: A dietary guide that encourages adequate nutrition and caloric intake.

Meta-analysis: A method of analysis that combines the results of a number of scientific studies, each addressing a related research hypothesis.

Metabolic rate: The rate of energy production in the body.

Mindfulness: A moment-to-moment awareness of one's thoughts, feelings, motivations, and actions. Mindfulness originated as a state of meditation within the Buddhist tradition.

Multidisciplinary: Two or more professional disciplines working collaboratively. In health care, it refers to delivery of services by professionals from a variety of healthcare specialties.

Muscle dysmorphia: A condition in which a person becomes fixated on the idea that he or she is not muscular enough and is inordinately preoccupied with thoughts concerning appearance, especially musculature.

N

Naso-gastric: A tube that is inserted through the nose or mouth and into the stomach.

Neuroimaging: Techniques that allow mapping of the structure or function of the brain.

Neurotransmitter: A chemical substance in the brain that facilitates communication between nerve cells.

Norepinephrine: A neurotransmitter in the brain that is involved in the regulation of sleep, arousal, mood, and response to stressful stimuli.

Nutrition counseling: Counseling designed to help patients enhance their understanding of healthy eating, learn a balanced approach to food, make and maintain dietary changes, and increase motivation to acquire and maintain a healthy weight.

O

Obsessive-compulsive disorder (OCD): A form of anxiety consisting of intense, persistent, recurrent, and disturbing thoughts, impulses, and repetitive behaviors.

Obsessive-compulsive personality disorder (OCPD): A pervasive pattern of preoccupation with orderliness, perfectionism, and mental and interpersonal control, at the expense of flexibility, openness, and efficiency.

Off-label use: The permissible use of a drug in ways other than what was originally sanctioned.

Osteopenia: A decrease in bone density that is less severe than in osteoporosis.

Osteoporosis: A condition characterized by a progressive decrease in body density. Osteoporosis produces dry, brittle bones that may easily crack or collapse.

P

Partial-syndrome anorexia: A pattern of disordered eating in which a patient reports symptoms such as marked dietary restriction, weight preoccupation, and purging, but which fail to meet all of the diagnostic criteria for anorexia nervosa.

Peak bone mass: The stage of growth at which bones have reached maximum density and strength.

Personality disorders: Enduring, pervasive, and inflexible patterns of behavior, thought, and interaction with others that cause significant functional impairment or distress.

Pica: A disorder characterized by the persistent eating of non-nutritive substances, such as dirt, clay, paper, or chalk.

Postmenarcheal: Having established menstruation.

Post-traumatic stress disorder (PTSD): A severe form of anxiety that may develop after experiencing a traumatic, life-threatening, or other very distressing situation. Symptoms can also develop after witnessing an event that involves a threat to another person.

Precipitating event: A triggering event that precedes and/or contributes to the development of an illness.

Prenatal: Occurring or existing before birth.

Pre-pubertal: Before the onset of puberty.

Protective factor: A characteristic that decreases a person's likelihood of developing an illness.

Psychiatric disorder: A recognized, diagnosable illness that results in the impairment of a person's cognitive abilities, emotional health, or interpersonal relationships; also called mental illness.

Psychotropic: A medication or agent that affects mental functioning or behavior.

Purging: Self-induced vomiting, misuse of laxatives, diuretics, or enemas.

R

Rebound water retention: Fluid retained by the body after discontinuing diuretic treatment.

Rectal prolapse: Protrusion of the rectum (the lowest part of the intestine) through the anal canal.

Registered dietitian: A qualified, trained, and credentialed expert in food and nutrition.

Risk factor: A characteristic that increases an individual's likelihood of developing an illness.

Rumination disorder: A disorder in which a person, usually a child, regurgitates partially digested food before rechewing the food or spitting it out.

S

Satiety: The feeling of fullness or satisfaction after eating.

Self-efficacy: The impression or judgment of one's own capabilities.

Self-esteem: Personal opinions, judgments, or feelings about oneself.

Self-image: An individual's perception of his or her own self.

Semi-starvation: The state of being partially or nearly starved.

Serotonin: A brain chemical thought to be important for regulating sleep, appetite, mood, and pain inhibition.

Sliding scale: A fee scale that fluctuates in response to a patient's income and cost-of-living.

Social phobia: An anxiety disorder that is characterized by a persistent, intense fear of being evaluated, judged, criticized or humiliated in social situations. These fears can be triggered by the real or imagined scrutiny by others. Social phobia can cause extreme distress and may be accompanied by severe blushing, sweating, tearfulness, trembling. nausea, or feelings of panic.

Somatic: Pertaining to the body.

Sub-clinical: The stage of development of an illness before symptoms are observed; or the presentation of symptoms of an illness that do not meet the full diagnostic criteria of an illness or condition.

Substance use disorders: Alcohol use, drug use, and/or abuse may also co-exist with anorexia.

Symptom: A sign or indication of a disorder, disease, or condition.

T

Tachycardia: Abnormally rapid heart rate.

Thin ideal: Cultural attitudes which imply that extreme thinness is a requisite for attractiveness. Such ideas may inadvertently promote unhealthy weight control methods in society-at-large by promoting conformity to an unrealistic "ideal" body shape and size.

Tolerance: Physical or psychological adaptation to the effects of a substance or action, requiring larger amounts to produce the same desired effects.

Trans fats: Fats that have been treated with hydrogen. Used in many processed foods in order to increase shelf life and flavor stability.

Transition care: The preparation and training provided to patients who will soon leave inpatient or residential treatment (also known as transition-phase treatment).

W

Withdrawal: Characteristic symptoms that occur after the cessation of long-term use, or the sudden discontinuation of a drug or habit-forming action.

Glossary

Index

Index

Index